W9-BFU-675

The Source® for Executive Function Disorders

by Susanne Phillips Keeley

GOVERNORS STATE UNIVERSITY LIBRARY

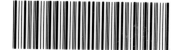

3 1611 00336 3873

Skill	Ages
■ executive functions	■ 16 through adult

Evidence-Based Practice

■ Executive functions are a group of cognitive skills localized in the frontal lobe structures. Deficits in executive functioning involve both discrete skills and the processes that control the use of these skills (Cicerone et al., 2000).

■ Executive function deficits, including weakness in the areas of self-awareness, goal setting, and strategic thinking, are often among the most debilitating problems following brain injury (ASHA, 2003).

■ In assessing and treating executive function deficits, it is important to collaborate with the patient in selecting goals, testing treatment hypotheses, identifying strategic compensations, and monitoring results (ASHA, 2003; Cicerone et al., 2000).

■ Effective intervention is measured by the reduction of supports needed by the individual with a disability (ASHA, 2003).

The Source for Executive Function Disorders incorporates these principles and is also based on expert professional practice.

References

American Speech-Language-Hearing Association (ASHA). (2003). *Rehabilitation of children and adults with cognitive-communication disorders after brain injury* [Technical Report]. Retrieved March 10, 2009 from www.asha.org/policy

Cicerone, K., Dahlberg C., Kalmar K., Langenbahn, D., Malec, J., Bergquist, T., et al. (2000). Evidence-based cognitive rehabilitation: Recommendations for clinical practice. *Archives of Physical Medicine & Rehabilitation, 81*(12), 1596-1615.

LinguiSystems®

LinguiSystems, Inc.
3100 4th Avenue
East Moline, IL 61244
800-776-4332

FAX: 800-577-4555
Email: service@linguisystems.com
Web: linguisystems.com

Copyright © 2003 LinguiSystems, Inc.

All of our products are copyrighted to protect the fine work of our authors. You may only copy the forms and activities as needed for your own use. Any other reproduction or distribution of the pages in this book is prohibited, including copying the entire book to use as another primary source or "master" copy.

GOVERNORS STATE UNIVERSITY
UNIVERSITY PARK
IL 60466

Printed in the U.S.A.

ISBN 10: 0-7606-0503-3
ISBN 13: 978-0-7606-0503-5

RC
387.5
.K446
2003

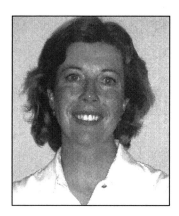

Susanne Phillips Keeley, M.S., CCC-SLP, earned degrees in Communication Disorders & Speech Science and Psychology from the University of Colorado. She received her M.S. in Speech-Language Pathology from Northwestern University and continues to work and live in the Chicago area.

She has specialized in the evaluation and treatment of adult neurological disorders in many settings, including inpatient acute care, outpatient, acute rehabilitation, home care, and private practice.

The Source for Executive Function Disorders is Susanne's first publication with LinguiSystems.

Dedication

To my parents, Betty and Jim, for their love; to my friends the Bradley Family, for their humor and encouragement and the Mates Family for their motivation and insight; to my husband, Bill, for his love and support; and to my children, Lauren and James, who make me smile every day.

Treatment

Comments to Therapists

The increasing prevalence of brain damage as a result of head trauma, stroke, or a tumor has resulted in a need for therapists skilled in the evaluation and treatment of this population. Materials developed for language-impaired individuals have not always been appropriate, and consequently, there has been an increase in the amount of commercially-available material targeting the brain-injured adult population. Most of these treatment manuals contain activities appropriate for levels of severity that range from mild to severe. Frequently, high-level assessments and treatment activities are mixed with lower-level tasks within the text. Often, they do not provide the comprehensive consideration the executive function disordered population requires. Using tasks designed for low-level patients and increasing the linguistic/attention/memory parameters of the task alone is not sufficient. Activities related to the patient's life and what the patient finds interesting are most likely to be effective. However, it is difficult to find specific task-training activities at the high level that could engage a patient for more than a few minutes, and certainly not an entire treatment course.

Because this book is devoted to rehabilitation practice, it assumes basic knowledge of neuroanatomy, neurophysiology, neurological disease/impairment, and the mechanisms of brain injury. It contains activities for both the therapist and the patient. It is based on the premise that the patient is the best interpreter of his or her particular impairment. It is the therapist's responsibility to ask the right questions in order to obtain this information, substantiate the complaint with evaluation tools, design treatment activities that address the deficit areas, and monitor progress. This manual provides a structured framework for therapists to guide the processes of evaluation and treatment of patients with executive function disorders.

Results of studies have illustrated the improvement of cognitive functioning via theoretically-based rehabilitation exercises that methodically target specific processes. *The Source for Executive Function Disorders* contains contrived, highly clinical activities systematically targeting specific processes. It goes the extra step, however, to assist the therapist in applying therapeutic remediation to activities in the patient's daily life. Of utmost importance is the therapist's ability to think and analyze. This manual will instruct the therapist in determining which areas and activities are appropriate for each individual client, the structured and systematic presentation of treatment stimuli, and important components of documentation.

Because of the high level of the activities necessary to treat patients with executive function disorders, the therapist must possess a certain level of skill with his or her own executive functions. For example, the therapist will be required to break down tasks into their component parts, train in methods of prioritization, and participate in difficult alternating and divided attention tasks. Just as not every speech-language pathologist has the "ear" to be a good voice therapist, without extra work and effort, not every therapist will fall into executive function treatment easily. Work through the activities in this manual yourself. Try them with your friends and family, and begin to develop a feeling for the wide range of normal.

Executive functions perform as a collective service that comes into play with all facets of cognitive processing.

What Are Executive Functions?

As one advances hierarchically through the animal chain, a larger portion of the brain's cortex is devoted to the frontal structures. This region of the brain is the most modern in evolutionary development, and it is the last to develop and mature in an individual.

The frontal lobes of the brain are marked by their neuroanatomic diversity. The frontal lobes have numerous connections to other sections of the brain, and the functions they carry out are the product of information collected from many locations in the central nervous system.

The frontal lobes are not only accountable for primary cognitive functions but also for coordinating and actualizing the activities involved in cognitive processing. The frontal lobes coordinate input from other sections of the brain, and they function to organize and regulate behavior necessary to reach accomplishment of certain tasks. The frontal lobes are fundamental to the executive functions of anticipation, goal selection, planning, self-monitoring, use of feedback, and completion of purposeful activities.

The anatomical positioning of the frontal lobes leaves them sensitive to injury. They rest against rough, bony protuberances of the inner, anterior skull and, as the result of head injury, are easily scratched or bruised. Damage to the frontal lobes results in a combination of behavioral and emotional deficits and cognitive problems—specifically, decreased executive functions.

9

Copyright © 2003 LinguiSystems, Inc.

Executive functions do not portray a single, distinct process. Instead, executive functions perform as a collective service that comes into play with all facets of cognitive processing. Executive functions are a collage of cognitive activities that encompass the ability to design actions toward a goal, to handle information flexibly, to realize the ramifications of behavior, and to make reasonable inferences based upon limited information. Additionally, executive functions can be thought of as encompassing such activities as anticipation, goal selection, planning, initiation of activity, self-regulation or self-monitoring, and use of feedback. The executive functions are detailed functions of logic, strategy, planning, problem solving, and reasoning.

Impairment of any or all of these executive functions may be present in spite of strong intellectual skills and unaffected language capacity. When executive functions are impaired, all other cognitive systems have the potential to be affected, even though those same systems may remain undiminished in isolation. Individuals with executive function impairments have difficulty with planning and organization. They are unable to identify what needs to be done and/or are unsure of how to accomplish the

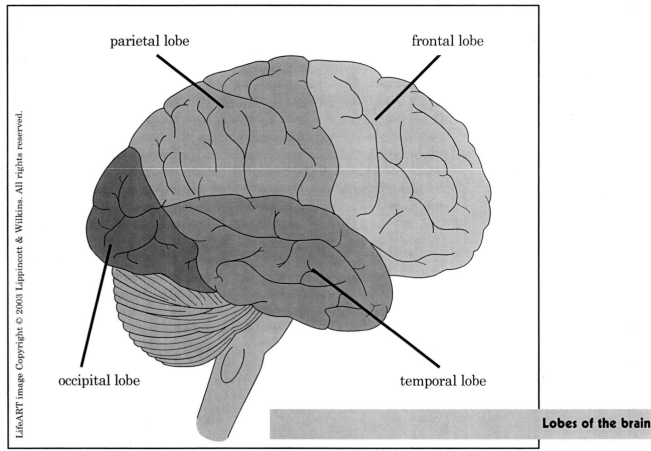

parietal lobe   frontal lobe

occipital lobe   temporal lobe

Lobes of the brain

LifeART image Copyright © 2003 Lippincott & Wilkins. All rights reserved.

Collecting the Patient History

The collection of information during the history section of the evaluation is an essential aspect of the assessment. By carefully questioning the patient and even more carefully listening to his or her answers, you can determine the areas to be assessed and treated. The patient history is not merely an opportunity to fill in the blanks on a form; instead, it is an opportunity to truly learn how the patient arrived at this point and how he or she hopes to be helped. Using the standard **Patient History** form on pages 21-24 allows the administrator to concentrate on the patient's answers and descriptions rather than formulating what question to ask next.

Helpful Hint: Fill out the history form while proceeding through the session. When appropriate, tape record or videotape the session to further allow for the opportunity to listen and respond.

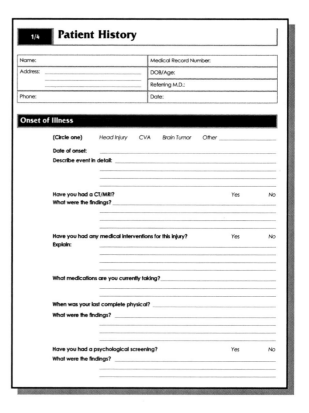

Onset of Illness

Collect the general demographic information and any facility-specific information. Begin by asking the patient to describe the injury/event in detail.

If this was an accident:

➤ Did the patient lose consciousness? If so, for how long? If not, did the patient feel "dazed"? How long did that feeling last? At what point did the patient begin to recall what was happening?

➤ Can the patient remember the events leading up to the accident? What about those after?

➤ Did a physician treat the patient? Was the patient hospitalized? For how long?

➤ Was a CT/MRI performed? If so, what were the results?

➤ Did the patient sustain any other injuries?

If this was a brain tumor:

➤ What symptoms led the patient to see a doctor in the first place?

➤ When was the patient diagnosed?

➤ Where was/is the tumor located? Does the patient know the type of the tumor?

➤ Did the patient have the tumor removed surgically?

➤ Has the patient had any radiation or chemotherapy?

➤ How have the symptoms changed during the course of medical treatment? Have any new symptoms appeared?

➤ Is the patient having routine CT/MRI scans? How often?

If this was a stroke:

➤ Did the patient have any symptoms prior to the stroke?

➤ What were the symptoms of the stroke?

➤ For how long did the stroke symptoms persist?

➤ Does the patient know what type of stroke it was or where it occurred in the brain?

➤ Is the patient receiving follow-up medical care since the stroke?

After gaining a clear understanding of the cause of the brain injury and medical intervention, obtain information regarding the patient's current medications. A number of drugs are implicated as causes of changed cognition. These include, but are not limited to, the medications listed on the following page.

- sedatives
- anticonvulsants
- antihypertensive drugs
- H2 receptor antagonists
- corticosteroids

- narcotics
- antidepressants
- anti-Parkinsonian drugs
- phenylthiazines

Helpful Hint: It is important to have a current *Physician's Desk Reference* handy. Call the patient's physician if you are unsure of a particular drug's possible affect on cognition.

During this phase of the examination, you should also ask the patient for details regarding alcohol consumption, drug abuse, over-the-counter medications, and vitamins or herbal supplements.

When was the patient's last complete physical? Despite being under a doctor's care for the brain injury, a general physical may not have been conducted. A variety of medical conditions can cause alterations in mental status and cognitive abilities. These include, but are not limited to, the following:

- hypertension
- cardiac illness
- vitamin B12 deficiency
- leukemias
- uremia
- hypercalcemia
- gypomagnesemia
- diabetes mellitus

- hypotension
- severe anemia
- sickle cell disease
- liver disorders
- hyper/hyponatremia
- hyperparathyroidism
- thyroid disorders
- nutritional disorders

- infectious diseases including Lyme disease and HIV infection

It is important that a medical physician be involved to rule out any medical conditions responsible for changed cognition. Refer the patient to his or her physician if he or she has not received a complete physical.

Of equal importance is the patient's psychological health. Brain injury, and specifically frontal lobe injury, can cause behavioral and emotional changes. Determine whether a psychological screening has been conducted to rule out anxiety, depression, or other psychological diagnoses that may be responsible or contributing to the changed condition. Refer the patient to a neuropsychologist or back to his or her physician if this has not been conducted.

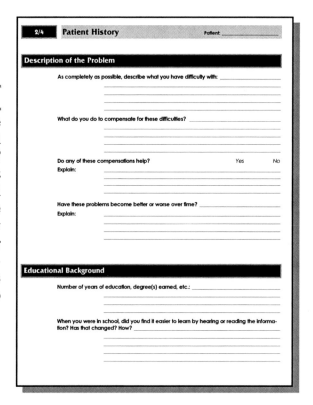

Description of the Problem

At this point in the interview, focus turns to the patient's complaint. What exactly does the patient find difficult or changed from his or her usual status? Patients know clearly what is challenging for them but do not always provide good descriptions. Most will require prompts to be more specific and to generate examples. It is the therapist's responsibility to narrow and clarify the scope of the patient's complaint. For example, if the patient states, "I can't remember anything!" the therapist follows with questions and cues such as those listed below and on the following pages to define this more distinctly.

Patient Comment	Clinician Follow-Up
I can't remember anything.	Give me an example of something you recently failed to remember.
	Do you have more trouble recalling information that you hear or that you read?
	Do you have more difficulty remembering "important" information or more casual, conversational information?
	Can you remember what you did yesterday?
	Can you remember what you are supposed to do this weekend?
	When you forget something, do you eventually remember or must you be reminded?
	Are there particular things you always have difficulty remembering?
I have trouble getting anything done.	Are you able to identify what tasks you want or need to accomplish?
	Do you have more difficulty completing simple daily tasks or long-term projects?
	Is it easy to generate the steps involved in completing the activity?

Patient Comment	Clinician Follow-Up
	Do you have trouble getting started?
	Are you easily drawn off task?
	Do you frequently feel overwhelmed with what needs to be accomplished?
I can't pay attention to anything.	Can you focus on something you are really interested in for 5-10 minutes? At what length of time do you lose attention in this interesting task?
	Can you concentrate in the midst of distractions?
	Can you do two things at one time?
	Do you "space out" and daydream or move on to another task? How long will this last?
	Are you aware of when you lose attention?
I'm always late.	Are you aware of when an event is scheduled?
	Are you conscious of the time during the day?
	Do you know how long it will take you to do something or get somewhere? What makes you late?

Helpful Hint: Asking the patient to provide examples can be very helpful in understanding the patient's complaint.

Does the patient utilize any compensatory strategies? What are these strategies and how successful are they? Pose questions (such as the following) to the patient in order to understand strategies and compensations being used.

➤ Does the patient use a calendar?
➤ Does the calendar have hour by hour slots, or is it for the whole day?
➤ How often does the patient look at the calendar?
➤ How consistent is the patient in writing in the calendar?
➤ Has the patient always used a calendar? Has the method of usage changed? Has the success with the calendar changed?
➤ Does the patient wear a watch? Always or recently?
➤ Does the patient keep lists? Is this a new behavior? If not, has the method changed?
➤ Does the patient turn off the TV or radio before starting to do something? Is this a new pattern?
➤ Does the patient limit activities to one at a time? Is this something new?
➤ Does the patient complete one task before moving on to the next?

Lastly, has the patient noted change in the deficits over time? Most patients will feel the problem has become worse. Perhaps it has, or perhaps the farther from "usual" the patient goes, the greater the frustration and feeling of decline. Again, the therapist's ability to clarify the issue is key.

Patient Comment	Clinician Follow-Up
I didn't have any problems right after the injury.	Did you return to work/school? Did you maintain your previous schedule?
	Did you maintain your previous responsibilities?
I was doing fine for a while.	Did you receive regular feedback from your supervisor, friends, or family?
	Were you receiving assistance from others at home/work?
	Do you feel you are expected to perform at "pre-injury" levels at this point?
I wasn't this tired before.	Were you keeping the same schedule as now?
	Are your medications the same?
	Were your responsibilities of the same level of difficulty as now?

Educational Background

Take the following questions into consideration when completing this section:

➤ How much schooling has the patient completed? Lower levels of education do not negate the existence of high-level deficits. Adults are required to be proficient in a large variety of attention, memory, and language skills, regardless of educational levels achieved; however, patients earning advanced degrees in mathematics should find no difficulty balancing a checkbook. Knowing the patient's premorbid level of education allows for assumptions about premorbid abilities.

➤ What subjects/topics were challenging for the patient in school? Have these areas continued to be challenging even outside the school setting? Everyone has strengths and weaknesses. Being aware of the patient's perceived areas of weakness assists in making realistic estimates of impairments.

➤ What was the patient's learning style during school? How did the patient learn and recall information while in school? Was the patient an auditory learner—able to recall the lectures more easily than the textbook—or vice versa? Does the patient feel this pattern of learning has continued? Does the patient feel this pattern of learning has changed as a result of the brain injury? Emphasize the preferred learning style during therapy whenever possible.

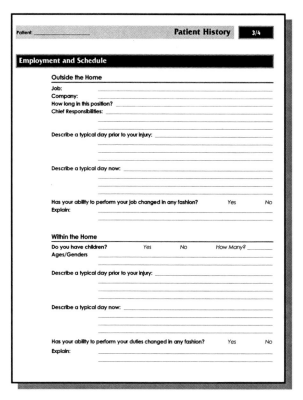

Employment and Schedule

At this point in the history collection, define the patient's work and home regimens. Ask the patient to describe, in detail, his or her work prior to the injury. The word *work* is intended in its broadest form: it is not limited to outside the home/office work. Women or men working in the home should proceed through the same descriptions and questioning. Ask the patient to portray a typical day. Ascertain the following from the patient:

➤ the time schedule of events/tasks
➤ the amount of tasks required in a day
➤ the type of tasks
➤ the dependence/independence upon others for completing the tasks
➤ the people available for assistance
➤ the number of people/number of tasks for which others depend upon the patient
➤ the physical surroundings (quiet or noisy, in an office or cubical, or in the open)
➤ whether the patient is in one location for the duration of the day or is required to move about
➤ the number and type of distractions and interruptions in the day
➤ whether each day is the same

Understanding the expectations of a "normal day" is fundamental to restoring the patient's routine.

Helpful Hint:	This task may also be used as a homework assignment encompassing written expression.

Complete the same line of questioning for a typical day since the injury. The therapist can complete the **Patient Comparison** chart on page 25 for pre- and post-injury to more easily see the variations.

Once treatment begins, the therapist's responsibility will be to analyze tasks the patient finds difficult and develop compensations/restoration techniques for these tasks. The more complete the therapist's understanding of the patient's life situation pre- and post-injury, the better the therapist will be in developing appropriate intervention tasks.

Past Medical History

Obtain past medical history information. Specifically, ask whether the patient has ever had previous head or brain injuries. This includes concussion, which the patient will likely not consider a head injury. Remember that brain injury is cumulative: the current injury may be compounded by previous minor incidences. Ask the patient about previous medications and the reason for their discontinuance. Perhaps the patient had a medical issue prior to the injury that may impact cognition and/or recovery. Determine whether there is or has been alcohol or substance abuse. Also, rule out or define previously diagnosed attention deficit disorder or learning disabilities. Ask whether the patient has any prior diagnosis/treatment for anxiety, depression, panic attacks, or other psychological diagnoses. Insure that the appropriate professionals are involved in treatment.

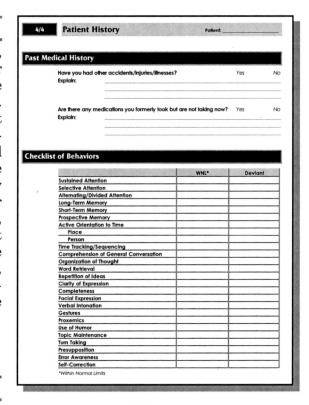

Checklists and Observations

In addition to obtaining facts during this initial discussion, you can collect information regarding the patient's ability to recall information, orient events in time, comprehend questions, express thoughts, comprehend and use nonverbal cues, and use pragmatics. Use the checklist as a cursory record of subjective observations. Deviancies will point toward areas requiring formal assessment.

Patient History

Name:	Medical Record Number:
Address: _____	DOB/Age:
_____	Referring M.D.:
_____	
Phone:	Date:

Onset of Illness

(Circle one)   *Head Injury*   *CVA*   *Brain Tumor*   *Other* _____

Date of onset: _____

Describe event in detail: _____
_____
_____
_____

Have you had a CT/MRI?   *Yes*   *No*

What were the findings? _____
_____
_____
_____

Have you had any medical interventions for this injury?   *Yes*   *No*

Explain: _____
_____
_____
_____

What medications are you currently taking?_____
_____
_____

When was your last complete physical? _____

What were the findings? _____
_____
_____
_____

Have you had a psychological screening?   *Yes*   *No*

What were the findings? _____
_____
_____

Description of the Problem

As completely as possible, describe what you have difficulty with: _____

_____

_____

_____

_____

What do you do to compensate for these difficulties? _____

_____

_____

_____

_____

Do any of these compensations help?   Yes   No

Explain: _____

_____

_____

_____

Have these problems become better or worse over time? _____

Explain: _____

_____

_____

_____

Educational Background

Number of years of education, degree(s) earned, etc.: _____

_____

_____

When you were in school, did you find it easier to learn by hearing or reading the information? Has that changed? How? _____

_____

_____

_____

_____

Employment and Schedule

Outside the Home

Job: _____

Company: _____

How long in this position? _____

Chief Responsibilities: _____

_____

_____

Describe a typical day prior to your injury: _____

_____

_____

_____

Describe a typical day now: _____

_____

_____

_____

Has your ability to perform your job changed in any fashion?   Yes   No

Explain: _____

_____

Within the Home

Do you have children?   Yes   No   How Many? _____

Ages/Genders _____

_____

Describe a typical day prior to your injury: _____

_____

_____

_____

Describe a typical day now: _____

_____

_____

_____

Has your ability to perform your duties changed in any fashion?   Yes   No

Explain: _____

_____

Past Medical History

Have you had other accidents/injuries/illnesses? Yes No

Explain: _____
_____
_____

Are there any medications you formerly took but are not taking now? Yes No

Explain: _____
_____
_____

Checklist of Behaviors

	WNL*	Deviant
Sustained Attention		
Selective Attention		
Alternating/Divided Attention		
Long-Term Memory		
Short-Term Memory		
Prospective Memory		
Active Orientation to Time		
Place		
Person		
Time Tracking/Sequencing		
Comprehension of General Conversation		
Organization of Thought		
Word Retrieval		
Repetition of Ideas		
Clarity of Expression		
Completeness		
Facial Expression		
Verbal Intonation		
Gestures		
Proxemics		
Use of Humor		
Topic Maintenance		
Turn Taking		
Presupposition		
Error Awareness		
Self-Correction		

*Within Normal Limits

Patient Comparison

Name:	Medical Record Number:	
Address: _____ _____ _____	DOB/Age:	
	Referring M.D.:	
Phone:	Date:	

	Pre-Injury	**Post-Injury**
Daily time schedule:		
➤ waking		
➤ sleeping		
➤ naps		
➤ appointments		
Amount of tasks required in a day		
➤ type of tasks		
Dependence/independence upon others for completing the tasks		
People available for assistance		
Number of people/number of tasks for which others depend upon the patient		
Physical surroundings; quiet or noisy, in an office or cubical, or in the open		
In one place for the duration of the day or required to move about		
Number and type of interruptions that occur in the day		
Is each day the same?		

Formal/Informal Assessment Tools

Once you've obtained the patient's history and description of the problem, evaluate these complaints, determine their severity, and compare against expected levels of performance. Standardized assessment instruments provide information about performance under controlled conditions. The patient's performance is compared to normative data on others with similar age and/or education. There are a variety of commercially-available, formal assessment procedures specifically designed for brain injury. Areas that are important to assess include:

- orientation
- attention
- short-term memory
- long-term memory
- prospective memory
- new learning
- word retrieval
- reading comprehension
- reading speed
- written content and organization
- mathematical accuracy and speed
- convergent reasoning
- divergent reasoning
- inductive reasoning
- deductive reasoning
- problem solving
- sequencing
- mental flexibility

Whenever a formal, normative test demonstrates the described deficit, it is the superior method of evaluation. Frequently however, neither the executive function deficit nor the severity of the deficit are highlighted via standardized instruments. Traditional standardized tests do not mirror the true demands that are made in everyday life. Adequate performance on a standardized test does not rule out executive function disorders. Instead, adjunctive modifications to the test or entirely new assessment methods must be utilized.

Non-standardized tasks provide a more functional picture of performance and offer a reflection of the patient's performance in real-life tasks. Non-standardized assessment allows for examining performance in different contexts and situations, which is a crucial component in executive functioning. There are several modifications to standardized tests that more effectively tap into executive functions. Formal assessment measures are carefully designed, and altering the stated design of the test negates the normative information. The patient can no longer be compared to other patients but can, nevertheless, be compared to himself or herself in a pre- and post-test fashion. There are several modifications to a standardized instrument or subtest that are beneficial in executive function assessment.

Modifications in Presentation

➤ *Order of Presentation:* Frequently, tests are structured in a hierarchical fashion with the most difficult items at the end of the test. When these later occurring items are in error, it is hard to determine whether the difficulty of the item was the key deterrent or whether it was the late presentation of the item challenging sustained attention. By presenting more difficult items first and proceeding to easier items, this question can be answered and assumptions made regarding sustained attention skills.

Another variation of presentation is to be truly random. Often patients "tune in" to a greater extent when they perceive tasks as difficult. Alternating between the more simple and more complex will eliminate the opportunity to establish a pattern of response.

➤ *Staged Interruptions:* To determine how the patient responds to interruptions, schedule a phone call, page, or door knock during the testing. Is the patient able to return easily to the task or does the patient require some time to "regroup"? The patient's response to the situation can provide information about alternating attention and the ability to start and stop tasks.

➤ *Distractions:* Most testing situations are ideal—a quiet, well-lit, well-heated/cooled clinical room. This is not how most life situations occur. Administer the assessment in a noisy environment with distracting activities surrounding the task. By doing this, you can judge the patient's selective attention (how easily the patient can tune out distractions and concentrate on the work at hand). Administer the same assessment or variation in a quiet testing environment for comparison.

Copyright © 2003 LinguiSystems, Inc.

➤ *Dual Assessment:* If the patient describes difficulty doing more than one thing at a time, mimic this in the assessment. Can the patient alternate between two subtests and maintain the same degree of accuracy as with a single task? Is the patient more able to alternate between two reading tasks vs. between a reading and a math task?

➤ *Time Constraints:* The perception of being hurried can impact performance. Telling the patient that there is a limited time to complete the task can impact performance. The actual imposition of these time constraints is optional.

➤ *Mix It Up:* Combine the above modifications. How does performance compare when the patient has less time to respond and is faced with distractions?

Modifications in Scoring

Standardized scoring methods of a formal assessment tool are only one method of determining performance. Other variables of the patient's performance should be considered and quantified. (When you've made modifications to the prescribed administration of the test you *must* modify scoring.)

➤ *Accuracy:* Most testing sections can be scored as number right vs. number wrong. This can be transformed into a percentage score.

➤ *Speed:* Timing how long a particular section, or the entire test, takes to complete can highlight those patients who have extended processing time. Conversely, some patients may complete tasks at a very quick pace. Compare how the patient's speed of performance changes relative to the modifications in presentation described previously.

➤ *Completeness:* With what degree of thoroughness did the patient complete the task? Deficits may be noted in skipping items, omitting details, and/or failing to complete the task. Document the percentage of items falling into these situations. On the other end of the spectrum, patients who have difficulty monitoring their output and ending tasks may generate far more than is necessary.

➤ *Efficiency:* Never set up an evaluation task and turn away. Note how the patient completes the task. Is it done in a logical, proficient manner, or is it attempted haphazardly? Document the method the patient uses to complete the task. Compare how the patient's efficiency varies relative to the modifications in presentation previously described.

➤ *Error Awareness:* Note if the patient spontaneously reviews his or her work or comments on errors during the testing. Allow the patient to "self-grade" the work. Can the patient identify errors? Document the percentage of errors the patient is able to identify independently and when given cues. Compare the patient's ability to identify errors when modifications in presentation are made.

➤ *Self-correction:* If error awareness is present, determine if the patient can expand this to correction. Is the patient able to correct spontaneously or are cues required? If you identify errors for the patient, can he or she correct them independently? Document the percentage of identified errors that the patient can self-correct. Compare the patient's ability to correct errors when modifications in presentation are made.

Life Task Simulation

Manipulating the methods of presentation and scoring of standardized evaluation tools is one method of evaluation. Additionally, observing the patient participating in tasks described as difficult is a beneficial evaluation tool.

Having determined a typical pre-injury day for the patient during the **Patient History** section of the evaluation, usual tasks for the patient have been identified. Simulate one of these tasks and quantify the patient's performance in terms of the modifications in scoring described previously. For example:

➤ Generate a typed memo regarding a hypothetical situation.
➤ Complete a form or check while requesting a phone number from information.
➤ Read a newspaper article with the radio on.
➤ Scan the TV schedule while talking on the phone.
➤ Complete a time card.
➤ Develop a shopping list from a specific recipe.
➤ Find the least expensive airfare from a newspaper ad, Internet service, or phone call.
➤ Sort 25 children into carpools for a hypothetical field trip.

Checklists and Questionnaires

Checklists and questionnaires are excellent tools to clarify patients' difficulties. They can also serve to quantify subjective complaints. A number can be assigned to each level of response. The scale below is used to complete the checklists on pages 31 and 32:

➤ Almost always = 5
➤ Usually = 4
➤ Sometimes = 3
➤ Seldom = 2
➤ Almost never = 1

This technique permits a numerical score to be attached to an item or group of items. Changes in the patient's rating as treatment commences can be reported as changes in score.

Copyright © 2003 LinguiSystems, Inc.

Patient Checklist 1

Name:	Medical Record Number:
Address: _____ _____	DOB/Age:
	Referring M.D.:
Phone:	Date:

	almost always	usually	sometimes	seldom	almost never
	5	**4**	**3**	**2**	**1**
I find it easy to determine my 2-3 priority tasks for the day.					
I find it easy to schedule my 2-3 important tasks for the day.					
I find it easy to know the steps involved in completing my 2-3 tasks.					
I accomplish my 2-3 tasks daily.					
I am efficient in completing tasks.					
I complete tasks by their deadline.					
I find it easy to get started on tasks and don't procrastinate.					
I find it easy to stop working on a task when it is time to do something else.					
I am not easily distracted from the activity at hand.					
I work on my difficult tasks when my energy is at its peak.					
Tasks typically take the amount of time I expect.					
I am able to modify my schedule when things don't go as planned.					
I don't delay difficult tasks.					
I never forget an appointment.					
I am on time and prepared for engagements.					
I return calls when I say I will.					
I complete projects in an organized fashion.					
I can see different ways to complete a task.					
I feel like I have enough mental energy during the day.					
My daily activities reflect and support my overall goal.					

Patient Checklist 2

Name:	Medical Record Number:
Address: _____	DOB/Age:
_____	Referring M.D.:
Phone:	Date:

	almost always	usually	sometimes	seldom	almost never
	5	**4**	**3**	**2**	**1**
I recall things I was told or did yesterday.					
I remember where things are kept.					
I remember to take belongings with me and not leave them behind.					
I remember to do what I said I would do.					
I remember details of my daily routine.					
I rarely retell a story or joke to the same person.					
I recall what I am supposed to do in the future (I keep my appointments).					
I recall stories I hear on the news.					
I recall stories I read in the paper.					
I can concentrate for long periods of time.					
I can ignore distractions.					
I can do two things at once.					
I have no difficulty coming back to something after an interruption.					
I rarely catch myself daydreaming.					
I rarely get so deeply involved in a task that I forget other obligations.					
I rarely get lost.					
I have no difficulty learning a new skill.					
I rarely feel confused.					
I find it easy to make decisions.					
I find it easy to pick up new skills.					

  Copyright © 2003 LinguiSystems, Inc.

Patient-Initiated Continuum (PIC)

In 1989, Lomas[1], et al., published a measure of functional communication for adult aphasics, *The Communicative Effectiveness Index (CETI)*. The *CETI* is a 16-item rating of communication situations allowing the individual with aphasia, a significant other, and the clinician an opportunity to judge the aphasic's functional communication[1].

The premise of the *CETI* can be modified to provide a patient-driven assessment and treatment tool via the *Patient-Initiated Continuum*, or *PIC*. *PIC* is a tool targeted to high-level cognitive and/or language impaired patients, as these patients have the greatest ability to understand their deficits and the impact these deficits have on daily functioning. (Three examples of completed *PIC*s are on pages 35-36.)

Methods

1. The patient is asked to identify 5-10 specific skills he or she feels are impaired and adversely affect daily performance at home and/or work. Frequently, patients require cues to generate highly specific items. For example, "I can't remember anything" would spur queries to determine if the patient was describing reductions in memory for material heard vs. read, immediate recall vs. delayed, familiar vs. novel, etc. With guidance from the therapist, the patient generates characteristics of his or her deficit and the functional impact.

2. These characteristics are next transcribed on paper in a landscape fashion with a 10-inch line drawn above each item. The far left-hand margin is labeled "Fully Unacceptable" and "Fully Acceptable" is written on the far right-hand margin.

[1]Lomas J., Pickard L., Bester S., Elbard H., Finlayson A., Zoghaib C. (1989). The communicative effectiveness index: development and psychometric evaluation of a functional measure for adult aphasia. *Journal of Speech and Hearing Disorders*, 54:113-124.

33
Copyright © 2003 LinguiSystems, Inc.

3. The patient is then asked to mark where on the continuum the patient feels his or her skills currently fall. Using a 10-inch line, the therapist can extrapolate these marks to percentages. For example, a mark at the 5½ inch point indicates that the patient perceives his or her performance to be 55% of personal expectation. (Note: the examples presented on pages 35-36 are shown at 50% of actual size.)

4. The patient will again rate his or her level on the continuum during and at the end of treatment, providing a visual and numerical comparison of progress.

Parameters of treatment can be fashioned from the deficits stated by the patient. The fact that the patient volunteered specific areas predisposes his or her interest in that area.

Summary

The *PIC*, used as an adjunct to formal assessment tools, provides several advantages:

➤ It actively involves the patient in understanding his or her impairment. It requires patients to put into daily terms what they find difficult, regardless of clinical test scores. The patient's ability or inability to verbalize specific areas of difficulty indicates the level of explanation and counsel needed to accompany treatment. For example, a patient who independently identified that material read is easier to recall than lectures does not require the same introduction and explanations as one who could not identify this difference.

➤ The *PIC* actively involves the patient in goal-setting. By participating in the *PIC*, the patient has shown what problems he or she notes and values as important to remedy. By comparing the *PIC* to formal test results, the therapist can prioritize which areas are impaired and which ones the patient wishes to address. Perhaps the patient scored poorly on an assessment of math yet never mentioned any math focus on the *PIC*. This is clearly not an area of priority to the patient.

➤ The *PIC* provides a comparison between perception and reality. Deviations between performance on formal test measures and the *PIC* can demonstrate how accurately the patient is able to judge his or her own performance. The *PIC* can also highlight the advantages or disadvantages a clinical testing situation provides.

➤ The *PIC* provides a method of quantifying patient performance and improvement. A percentage or number score can be assigned to each mark on the continuum. Patients serve as their own control; therefore, a therapist can report that the patient improved from an initial assessment to discharge assessment on a particular goal by a quantified amount.

34

Copyright © 2003 LinguiSystems, Inc.

PIC Example 1

Fully Unacceptable				Fully Acceptable
	X			

Remembering work schedule in my head

	X			

Remembering family/social schedule in my head

		X		

Budgeting my time well at work

	X			

Staying on track with the priorities I do set — maintaining focus

			X	

Bluntness in communication

	X			

Indecisiveness in social decisions

PIC Example 2

Fully Unacceptable				Fully Acceptable
		X		

Ability to use vocabulary desired

	X			

Ability to know/recall/keep appointments

	X			

Ability to reschedule from memory

X				

Ability to organize self better in the mornings to get out of house (not sidetracked)

	X			

Ability to finish one task before beginning another

			X	

Ability to SEE what is in front of me when I look

PIC Example 3

Fully Unacceptable		Fully Acceptable

X

Thinking at a reasonable speed

X

Focusing attention for reading

X

Being on time for appointments

X

Telling a story concisely and purposefully

X

Remembering details from meetings

X

Focusing attention for the entire meeting

Reports and Documentation

The use of standardized and informal assessment tools is the determinant of the presence or absence of executive function disorders.

➤ Are the patient's complaints consistent with executive function disorders?

➤ Are these complaints demonstrated via normative data?

➤ Are these complaints demonstrated via quantified informal assessment?

➤ Can these deficits be attributed to any other physical and/or psychological cause?

Documenting findings and developing appropriate long- and short-term goals are key, not only to successful treatment, but also for reimbursement and developing a referral base. Each facility will have its own method for documentation; however, several sections should be included.

History

This section includes a summary of the information gained during the interview with the patient and any accompanying medical reports. It includes the nature and severity of the injury, medical conditions, and medical treatment. It also will include the patient's educational and occupational situation and his or her complaint. The history section of the report establishes the medical indications for the referral.

This 37-year-old male was involved in a motor vehicle accident on 4/1/03. He does not report any loss of consciousness. He was treated in the emergency department of his local hospital. CT and MRI scans were negative. Since returning to work he reports difficulty in concentrating. He finds himself easily distracted. He reports missing appointments and forgetting engagements. He has been examined by a neurologist. A repeat CT demonstrated mild frontal lobe involvement bilaterally. Mr. B is a high school graduate who has been employed for 10 years as a supervisor of over 20 people. He does not take any medications on a regular basis and denies any alcohol or drug abuse.

Ms. S, a 60-year-old female, was diagnosed with a left frontal meningioma 3 months ago after suffering a seizure. She underwent a craniotomy and resection. No radiation or chemotherapy was recommended. All follow-up exams have been unremarkable. Ms. S complains that since the surgery she "does not feel like doing anything." She has not returned to her leisure activities and reports frequently failing to grocery shop and pay bills. Ms. S is a widowed homemaker with 2 grown children and 4 grandchildren who live nearby. She is currently taking Dilantin and denies alcohol or drug use.

Subjective

This section allows the therapist to offer subjective, yet clinical, observations regarding the patient and his or her response to the testing environment. For example:

- ➤ Did the patient arrive on time to the appointment?
- ➤ Was the patient's appearance consistent with expectations?
- ➤ Was the patient able to attend to the questions?
- ➤ Did the patient answer questions in a concise or haphazard manner?
- ➤ Did the patient have a good understanding of his or her deficits?
- ➤ Could the patient attend to the assessment?
- ➤ Were breaks required?
- ➤ Did the patient require frequent redirection?
- ➤ How did the patient respond to difficult tasks?

Subjectively, the patient appeared anxious about the testing situation. He verbally stated that he was nervous and displayed nervousness throughout the session. He was slow to respond throughout the session. He appeared to take a great deal of time to think through each response, even those that should be fairly automatic. Mr. B requested several breaks within the 1-hour session. He was, however, able to understand and carry out instructions without repetitions.

Ms. S arrived 15 minutes late for her scheduled appointment. She reported getting lost even though she is familiar with this building. Ms. S appeared disheveled in her appearance. She did not accept any suggested breaks during the assessment session even when she had obviously lost her attention to the task. It was difficult for her to maintain attention to a task or conversation for more than 5 minutes. When finished, Ms. S had difficulty locating her schedule book and requested to call later to schedule the next session. After 3 days she had not called and was therefore recontacted. At that time, she expressed her frustration at forgetfulness and scheduled the next appointment.

Test Score Reporting

Name:	Medical Record Number:
Address:	DOB/Age:
	Referring M.D.:
Phone:	Date:

Test Name	Number Correct	Percentile for Age
QRST	15/30 = 50%	43rd
1234	12/20 = 60%	38th
XYZ	4/10 = 40%	30th

Results

This part of the report contains specific test scores. These are easy to report in a table/grid format, such as the one provided on page 43 and pictured here.

Non-standardized scores are more difficult to report in a table format and frequently require more description. For example,

The patient was able to read a complete newspaper article (8 paragraphs) and answer questions regarding its content; however, this took over 15 minutes. When the patient was required to read the entire article in 5 minutes, performance dropped such that only 3 paragraphs were complete and accuracy of information for those 3 paragraphs was 55%.

When asked to check his own work, Mr. B was unable to identify any errors. When errors were pointed out to him, he was successful in making corrections.

When the most difficult portions of the test were administered first, the patient performed well on these. Her performance declined over time despite the declining level of difficulty.

The **Results** section will also include functional statements regarding the patient's performance in daily tasks. For example,

Functionally, he comprehended and participated in adult conversation in the therapy room without difficulty. He recalled specifics and details of a general conversation without difficulty. When conversation was moved to a noisy environment, he had difficulty recalling even the main point of the conversation several minutes later. He expressed himself in complete, adult-level sentences with only occasional instances of word retrieval difficulties. His reading and writing were also at adult levels when conducted in a quiet environment. He had difficulty recalling the main point of a newspaper he scanned in the waiting room. In all conversation he appeared deliberate, as if it was difficult for him to maintain this level of performance. He showed

Copyright © 2003 LinguiSystems, Inc.

decline in all aspects of attention, both in the testing situation and in conversation. He was fairly accurate in identifying instances of reduced attention in this setting, frequently stating, "I'm not getting it." He often lost his train of thought. His awareness of this was fairly good, but his ability to self-correct was limited.

Functionally, Ms. S showed adequate focused and sustained attention for general conversation and for specific testing items. Despite this, she frequently complained that her "mind wants to be somewhere else." She did show reductions in divided and alternating attention both during structured testing and informal observation. She had a great deal of difficulty with tasks that required her to perform 2 functions simultaneously or alternate between 2 tasks. This was also noted in non-testing situations. Her ability to focus her attention in a distracting environment showed a significant reduction relative to her skill in a non-distracting environment.

Interpretation

Assigning a severity level to the executive function disorder, based on functional skills, is helpful in gradating the problem and judging improvement.

Severe — Profound difficulties resulting in an inability to perform daily functions for home and/or work tasks. Inability to successfully use compensatory strategies.

Moderately Severe — Inconsistent ability to generate and select appropriate goals, sequence the steps involved, and evaluate performance. Emerging ability to utilize compensatory strategies. Performance at home and work continue to be inconsistent.

Moderate — Consistent ability to generate and select goals and sequence the steps involved for 1-2 tasks. Difficulties in time management, speed of response, and evaluation of performance are present. Skills dramatically decline with increasing numbers of tasks. The use of compensatory strategies is consistent, but it is not comprehensive.

Mild-Moderate — Consistent ability to generate and select goals and sequence the steps involved and develop appropriate time references for multiple tasks. Speed of response and self-evaluation continue to show deficits. Use of compensatory strategies is consistent.

Mild — Ability to operate at home and work using compensatory strategies. Difficulties in multiple task organization, high-level organization, speed of response and behavioral self-management continue to be evident.

Minimal   Ability to perform most all tasks necessary for home
                            and work via compensatory techniques.

Goals

Goals of treatment must be:
> quantifiable
> measurable
> functional
> attainable

Each patient will have an entirely different set of long- and short-term goals specific to his or her particular needs. Identify areas of deficit based upon the results of both formal and informal testing. Determine what clinical parameters are involved in the patient's *PIC* responses. For instance, Example 1 on page 35 stated "Remembering family/social schedule in my head" as the patient's least acceptable item. Does the patient even know his or her schedule? Is it a realistic schedule? Is the schedule written down? Have any attempts at memorization been made, or is it expected to be automatic? Example 2 on page 35 stated "Ability to organize self better in the mornings to get out of the house (not sidetracked)" as most problematic. Goals for this patient would include establishing realistic schedules and routines and improving selective attention. Example 3 on page 36 listed "Focusing attention for the entire meeting" as the patient's biggest difficulty. Focus on sustained attention would be an important goal for the patient to meet.

The therapist and the patient must mutually agree upon goals, and this agreement must be documented in the report.

> **Long-term goals** are those to be accomplished over the course of treatment. They are functional and are the "end-product" of treatment. Here are some examples:
>   • *Consistent ability to identify necessary tasks for the day*
>   • *Consistent ability to sequence tasks and components of tasks*
>   • *Consistent ability to prioritize activities of the day*
>   • *Consistent ability to anticipate time constraints and requirements*
>   • *Consistent ability to modify plans based upon new information*
>   • *Attention skills adequate to participate in 30 minutes of adult conversation in a noisy environment*
>   • *Attention skills adequate to read for 30-40 minutes with adequate comprehension and retention*
>   • *Reading of an adult-level newspaper article, 8-10 paragraphs, in 5 minutes with adequate comprehension and retention*
>   • *Written production of 1-2 pages of adult level information with appropriate vocabulary and syntax, produced within 15 minutes*

Patients with executive function disorders must employ a great many compensatory strategies during their treatment, and often throughout life. They must be cognizant of these strategies and their uses. The therapist will develop and instruct in the use of compensations but the patient must know and use them. Therefore, long-term goals will be reflective of this. Here are some examples:

- *Consistent knowledge and use of compensatory strategies to improve attention*

- *Consistent knowledge and use of compensatory strategies to improve memory*

- *Knowledge of and independent use of an organizational system to manage time*

➤ **Short-term goals** are more clinical. They are specific tasks utilized in order to meet long-term goals. Their relationship to the long-term goals must be evident. Do not assume that the referring physician or the payer understands the correlation between visual scanning tasks and attention. Short-term goals are typically established for a 3-4 week duration. Specific performance criteria should be stated along with the cues, if any, needed to achieve this level. Here are some examples of short-term goals:

- *Ability to define 5 techniques to improve memory and the ability to use these techniques in treatment tasks when provided with an initial cue to do so*

- *Ability to state 2 strategies to maximize selective attention and the ability to use them consistently in clinical situations*

- *90% accuracy in paper and pencil tasks requiring alternating and divided attention*

- *90% accurate ability to complete simple pen and paper tasks with competing auditory stimuli*

- *Ability to sustain attention to reading of 3-4 paragraphs of adult level material interesting to the patient with 85% accuracy answering questions about the passage 15 minutes later*

- *Ability to accurately proofread 1 page of written material and make corrections*

- *Consistent ability to record time and date of therapy appointments in the patient's organizational system*

- *Accurate time estimations, within 10 minutes, for 10 activities within the patient's day*

Test Score Reporting

Name:		Medical Record Number:
Address:	_____	DOB/Age:
	_____	Referring M.D.:
	_____	
Phone:		Date:

Test Name	Number Correct	Percentile for Age

Comments _____

_____

_____

_____

_____

_____

_____

General Treatment Guidelines

Collecting the patient history and description of the complaint provided the blueprint for conducting the evaluation. Thorough evaluation via formal and informal measures confirmed and quantified the executive function disorders. The evaluation results provided a template to develop mutually determined goals for treatment. Working through systematic activities to achieve these goals is the next step.

Here are some general guidelines for planning treatment:

➤ Appreciate how the impairment aimed at remediation affects a patient's ability to understand, integrate, and retain information.

➤ Simplify the information provided. Try to use the patient's wording.

➤ Provide multiple trials, a slowed rate of presentation, well-organized written summaries and assignments, and session summaries.

➤ Be an active listener. Hear what the patient is saying and plan/modify the treatment based upon this active listening. Don't be so intent on completing your plan that you miss a perfect opportunity to address another goal in a meaningful way.

Metacognitive Processes

In the course of treatment, patients will be instructed to think about *how* they think. The patient will need to gain knowledge about cognitive processes, and through treatment, the patient will be assisted in developing or rediscovering strategies.

What exactly is a *strategy*? It is a tool, plan, or method used for accomplishing a task. As patients develop strategies they will:

➤ learn that there is more than one right way to accomplish a task.

➤ be able to identify their mistakes and try to rectify them.

➤ evaluate their end results.

In order to successfully instruct the patient in the use of strategies, the therapist should follow these steps:

1. **Describe the strategy.** Allow the patient to obtain an understanding of the strategy and its purpose: why it is important, when it can be used, and how to use it.

2. **Model the strategy's use.** Utilize the strategy during treatment sessions, providing direct models of the strategy, and explaining to the patient how to use the strategy in the particular situation.

3. **Provide practice tasks.** Provide the patient with opportunities to practice using the strategy in both functional and clinical tasks. Provide cues and feedback on the appropriate and accurate use of the strategy.

4. **Promote self-monitoring and evaluation.** Patients will use the strategy if they see how it assists them in meeting their goals.

The challenge in all therapy is for the patient to transfer and utilize the skills mastered during treatment sessions and structured activities in his or her everyday life. Carryover is a topic traditionally reserved for the end of treatment; however, the end product of therapy must be considered from the first day of involvement with the patient. Transfer is not automatic and must be addressed from the onset. Factors that influence generalization include the following:

➤ the degree to which the patient has attained automatic mastery of the skill

➤ an understanding of when the skill may be useful

➤ knowing how to modify the skill to fit different situations

➤ confidence and knowledge that the skill will be useful and successful in different situations.

Achieving carryover is most easily achieved by utilizing everyday situations throughout therapy. Occasionally, highly clinical, contrived tasks are necessary to train a skill, but the functional, daily application of that skill and task must be clear to the patient.

Self-Assessment

The ability to anticipate performance, accurately judge correct performance, and make modifications for future performance addresses the executive function disorder characteristics of self-regulation and use of feedback. Prior to completing tasks during treatment sessions and as homework, provide the patient with a copy of the **Performance Checklist** on page 48. Ask the patient to complete the first shaded column of the checklist (Predicted Performance Rating) using the following scale:

> **7** = I can complete this activity accurately and independently.
>
> **6** = I can complete this activity accurately with minimal cues.
>
> **5** = I can complete over half of this activity accurately and independently.
>
> **4** = I can complete over half of this activity accurately, given cues.
>
> **3** = I can complete less than half of this activity accurately and independently.
>
> **2** = I can complete less than half of this activity, given cues.
>
> **1** = I cannot complete this activity accurately, even with cues.

At the completion of the task, have the patient complete the second shaded column and the far right-hand column of the **Performance Checklist** to judge actual performance on the task(s). The ability to develop an accurate self-perception is an important element of executive functions.

Performance Checklist

Name:	Medical Record Number:
Address: _____ _____ _____	DOB/Age:
	Referring M.D.:
Phone:	Date:

Directions for Completing the Checklist

1. Describe the task in the first column.
2. Use the Rating Scale to the right to predict how well you will perform on the task.
3. Do the task.
4. Use the Rating Scale to the right to record your actual performance on the task.
5. Note the variance between your prediction and your actual performance, and provide any reasons for the variance.

Rating Scale

7 I can complete this activity accurately and independently.

6 I can complete this activity accurately with minimal cues.

5 I can complete over half of this activity accurately and independently.

4 I can complete over half of this activity accurately, given cues.

3 I can complete less than half of this activity accurately and independently.

2 I can complete less than half of this activity, given cues.

1 I cannot complete this activity accurately, even with cues.

Task	Predicted Performance Rating	Actual Performance Rating	Variance/Reason

Time Management

One of the skill deficits of executive function disorders is the inability to properly manage time. Time management includes the ability to understand, be aware of, and regulate activity according to time constraints.

There are four divisions of time management:
- **Time estimation:** the ability to judge the passage of time in general, and the ability to judge how long completion of a task will take
- **Time schedules:** the capability to generate an accurate and realistic time schedule
- **Completion of scheduled activities:** the ability to execute tasks in accordance with time schedules
- **Alterations:** the capacity to modify the schedule when new information is presented or when the original plan goes awry

Helpful Hint: Knowledge about time management can be found in many forms. The information provided in business publications is often more appropriate than that typically found in therapy publications. Make it a habit to walk through the business section in the library and read magazines pertaining to work habits and time management.

Everyone has variable time management abilities. Many people, including those without any documented injury, have difficulty arriving on time to events, planning an appropriate number of activities in a day, and/or altering their plans. While not expecting all patients to become scheduling wizards, imposing some form of structure on these divisions of time is key.

49

Copyright © 2003 LinguiSystems, Inc.

External System

Using an external time management system is an excellent starting point for the patient with executive function disorders. There are many commercially-available time management systems. Traditional black three-ring binder "memory books" are not typically appropriate with this population. If the patient already uses a particular system, allow the patient to continue with this system, making necessary modifications.

Helpful Hint: If the patient is not accustomed to external organization and time management tools, you will need to expose him or her to the options. Maintain examples and/or catalogs for various time management systems, such as DayPlanner, Filofax, Franklin Planners, and Palm Pilots. Learn the pros and cons of each.

The system must be large enough to hold the required information but small enough to be carried at all times. It should be used for both home and work activities. These elements must be included:

- ➤ full month calendar
- ➤ daily pages with time slots
- ➤ "to do" section
- ➤ daily log or diary section
- ➤ blank pages

The only system that will work is one that the patient will actually use. It is important that the patient be responsible for selecting a tool that fits his or her style. Once the patient has selected a system, begin by introducing and structuring the use of the system in measurable steps. The patient will need to bring his or her calendar system to every session, and ultimately, throughout all daily encounters. Treatment tasks and homework will focus on working through the steps needed to master the system, and thus, provide retraining and compensation for deficits in the four divisions of time management. Each patient will work through these treatment phases at a different pace. Some phases can easily be completed during therapy sessions, and some are more appropriately given for homework. They are cumulative. Once the patient has completed a phase during a session and/or for homework, you should continually check and evaluate this phase to establish a habitual nature.

Phase 1: Engraved in Stone

During the initial sessions of treatment and for homework, use the full month and daily calendars to have the patient enter all birthdays, anniversaries, and holidays (any events that will not change).

Helpful Hint: If national and religious holidays are not pre-established in the calendar system, cue the patient to fill these in also.

Sunday	Monday	Tuesday	Wednesday	Thursday	Friday	Saturday
1	2	3	4	5 Lauren Birthday	6	7
8	9	10	11	12	13	14 James Birthday
15	16	17 Mom & Dad Anniversary	18	19	20	21
22	23	24	25	26	27 Pay Day	28
29	30 Holiday	31				

	OCTOBER 5	Lauren Birthday
8:00		
9:00		
10:00		
11:00		
12:00		
1:00		
2:00		
3:00		
4:00		
5:00		
6:00		
7:00		
8:00		

Documentation:
- ➤ What percentage of recurring items were entered into the calendar?
- ➤ What percentage were on both the monthly calendar and the daily calendar?
- ➤ How many and what type of cues were required to achieve this level of accuracy?
- ➤ What type of errors were produced?

Phase 2: Scheduled Events

Once the "engraved in stone" items have been successfully accounted for, have the patient enter all scheduled appointments and events in the appropriate time slot on the appropriate day. Anything that must be done at a particular time should be included:

Helpful Hint:	For some schedules, entering all information in the monthly calendar section may be too crowded. Work to determine which appointments should be listed on both the monthly and the daily schedule.

- ➤ Begin with already scheduled doctor and dentist appointments.
- ➤ Enter all regularly occurring meetings.
- ➤ Enter all regularly occurring activities.

Example (New items are in **boldface** in all examples.):

Sunday	Monday	Tuesday	Wednesday	Thursday	Friday	Saturday
1	2	3 **9:00 Meet with Bob** **12:00 Lunch** **6:00 Meeting**	4	5 Lauren Birthday	6	7
8	9	10	11 **10:00 DDS**	12	13	14 James Birthday
15	16 **12:00 Jan Lunch**	17 Mom & Dad Anniversary	18	19	20	21
22	23	24	25	26	27 Pay Day	28 **8:00 Party**
29	30 Holiday **2:30 Picnic**	31				

	OCTOBER 3
8:00	
8:30	Meet with Bob
9:00	
10:00	
11:00	
12:00	Lunch at Main Street
1:00	
2:00	
3:00	
4:00	
5:00	
6:00	Meeting at Club
7:00	Dinner

Helpful Hint: Many patients are hesitant to relinquish appointment cards or "sticky notes" in favor of writing all information into the calendar. Consider incorporating an envelope into the organizational book to keep these cards.

Once events that have already been scheduled are entered on the calendar, begin to train the patient to consistently enter all new appointments and obligations directly into the calendar.

At each session, review the calendar:
- Ask patients whether they carry the calendar with them everywhere.
- Have any appointments, obligations, parties, meetings, etc., been scheduled since the last treatment session?
- Have these new events been documented in the calendar system?
- Are the events documented in the appropriate location?

Documentation:
- What percentage of appointments/events were written down?
- How many were not written down correctly?
- What kept the patient from entering the correct information consistently?
- Was there a pattern to the errors?
- What type of cues assisted the patient in improving his or her accuracy?

Now that those appointments and obligations determined by others have been accounted for, it's time to fill in the remainder of the tasks needed for each day.

Phase 3: Time Estimation

Estimating the time necessary to complete tasks is imperative and typically an area where patients develop an impasse. The patient may grossly over or underestimate the length of time a task requires. Making this mistake throughout the day can result in being hours off in scheduling. Over time, these hours translate into being days and weeks off schedule.

Prior to successfully slotting activities into appropriate time frames, provide the patient with practice judging the amount of time particular activities take to complete. For homework, provide the patient with a copy of the **Time Estimation Worksheet** on page 72 and have him or her follow these directions:

➤ Complete a simple table comparing the length of time the patient estimated a task would take to the actual time it took to complete.

➤ Carry out this exercise for a large variety of tasks (getting dressed, making phone calls, driving to appointments, shopping, etc.).

➤ Carry out this exercise for a number of days.

Analyze the table with the patient during a session. Consider the number of tasks where needed time was over or underestimated. Does the patient have an explanation for any discrepancies? Is there a pattern to the patient's errors, such as morning vs. afternoon tasks, physical vs. mental tasks, etc.

Helpful Hint:	Complete the **Time Estimation Worksheet** yourself and ask your friends to do so. Everyone is off in their estimations a bit. Develop a sense of what is a normal fluctuation as opposed to impaired ability.

The patient should continue with this exercise until his or her ability to accurately estimate the durations of tasks has been achieved. A completed example of a portion of the **Time Estimation Worksheet** is shown below. Tasks and activities that are appropriate for this activity include the following:

➤ showering or getting ready in the morning

➤ driving to work, school, or regular locations

➤ grocery shopping

➤ reading the newspaper

➤ making a meal

➤ changing sheets on a bed

➤ washing the dishes

➤ cleaning a room

➤ mowing the grass

➤ writing a letter or report

Task	Estimate	Actual
Shower	5 min.	10 min.
Drive to Store	10 min.	10 min.
Make Dinner	20 min.	35 min.
Do Dishes/Clean Up	10 min.	15 min.
Talk with Mom	10 min.	5 min.

Include additional activities specific to the patient's needs and daily routines.

54

Copyright © 2003 LinguiSystems, Inc.

Documentation:
➤ How many minutes or hours were over/underestimated?
➤ Was there a pattern to the errors?
➤ Were physical tasks more consistently miscalculated compared to mental?
➤ What percentage of activities were correctly estimated?

Once the patient has a good feel for how long tasks take, begin to calculate how many hours of the day are consumed by daily routines, work, chores, and other activities.

Phase 4: How Many Hours in a Day?

There are only so many hours in a day. Patients with executive function disorders have difficulty planning realistic schedules. They need to understand that every slot on the time grid cannot be filled with activity. Patients need help planning for both the incidentals and necessities in the day.

Walk the patient through the exercise of recognizing available time in the day. Have the patient complete a **Time Available Equation** on page 73. This mathematical exercise will visually demonstrate both the number of hours in a day that are consumed by already established activities and the "free," available time remaining.

Begin with 24 hours, and consider the following:
➤ How many hours does the patient sleep? Is the patient cheating his or her sleep to make more time in the day?
➤ Has the patient allotted time to eat? Again, patients often view this as a negotiable activity to steal more time. At the minimum, 3 meals will take 30 minutes of the day.
➤ Is the patient responsible for making these meals? How long does that take? What about the cleanup?
➤ Within the calculation, consider that it is typical to spend another half hour of each day, minimum, on miscellaneous activities such as getting a drink, using the bathroom, wasting a minute or two here or there, etc.
➤ How long does the patient's morning routine take? Evening/bedtime routine?

Next consider activities specific to the patient beyond sleeping, eating, and hygiene. This list will be particular to the patient. Patients often have difficulty coming up with such tasks on their own. Anticipate what obligations the patient may have and query the patient to determine what is included in the **Time Available Equation**. Here are some questions you might ask the patient:
➤ Do you commute?
➤ Are there standing commitments/obligations that take time?
➤ Do you drive others/children to school or various activities?

➤ Are you responsible for household duties such as washing, shopping, cooking, and cleaning?

Have the patient generate a list of time commitments, estimate the length of time needed to to accomplish each, and begin to subtract those periods from the 24-hour baseline. The top example on this page is based on a 24-hour day and the bottom example is a work setting equation that reflects a typical 40-hour work week.

The person who completed these equations found that he had just 5 available hours at home every day and 7.5 "free" hours at work each week. Typically, what is discovered by this exercise is the patient's unrealistic expectation of how many hours are available in any given day to complete individual obligations. This **Time Available Equation** should be thought of as an ongoing process that the patient evaluates frequently.

During this activity, the concept of *planning* should be introduced. Emphasize to patients that *a half hour of planning will save one hour of wasted time.*

Often, the pressure of having too much to do results in diving into the day without proper organization. It is essential that patients with executive function disorders come to understand and believe that this half hour planning time is necessary for success. This 30 minutes of planning should be reflected in the time available calculations, reducing the available time in the home example above to 4.5 available hours in a day and to 5 hours a week in the work example (30 minutes every day for 5 work days).

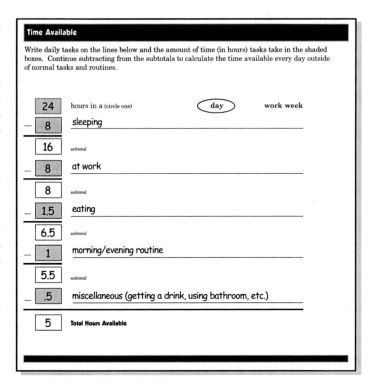

Time Available

Write daily tasks on the lines below and the amount of time (in hours) tasks take in the shaded boxes. Continue subtracting from the subtotals to calculate the time available every day outside of normal tasks and routines.

24	hours in a (circle one) ⟨day⟩ work week
− 8	sleeping
16	*subtotal*
− 8	at work
8	*subtotal*
− 1.5	eating
6.5	*subtotal*
− 1	morning/evening routine
5.5	*subtotal*
− .5	miscellaneous (getting a drink, using bathroom, etc.)
5	**Total Hours Available**

Time Available

Write daily tasks on the lines below and the amount of time (in hours) tasks take in the shaded boxes. Continue subtracting from the subtotals to calculate the time available every day outside of normal tasks and routines.

40	hours in a (circle one) day ⟨work week⟩
− 5	scheduled meetings
35	*subtotal*
− 10	writing
25	*subtotal*
− 10	on the phone
15	*subtotal*
− 5	unscheduled meetings, questions, etc.
10	*subtotal*
− 2.5	miscellaneous (getting a drink, using bathroom, etc.)
7.5	**Total Hours Available**

	OCTOBER 3
6:00	**Wake and Shower**
7:00	**Eat Breakfast**
8:00	**Planning**
8:30	Meet with Bob
9:00	
10:00	
11:00	
12:00	Lunch at Main Street
1:00	
2:00	
3:00	
4:00	
5:00	**Organize for Tomorrow**
6:00	Meeting at Club
7:00	Dinner

What about the time requirements before and after each activity? Does the patient allow for travel time or preparation time? This lack of planning contributes to tardiness and the constant feeling of being "behind" that patients with executive function disorders express. Help the patient to adequately schedule time for travel and preparation.

	OCTOBER 3
6:00	Wake and Shower
7:00	Eat Breakfast
7:30	**Leave for Work**
8:00	Planning
8:30	Meet with Bob
9:00	
10:00	
11:00	
11:30	**Drive to Lunch**
12:00	Lunch at Main Street
1:00	**Drive Back from Lunch**
2:00	
3:00	
4:00	
5:00	Organize for Tomorrow
5:30	**Drive to Meeting**
6:00	Meeting at Club
7:00	**Drive Home**
7:30	**Dinner**

57

Copyright © 2003 LinguiSystems, Inc.

Documentation:
➤ What percentage of total time-consuming activities was the patient able to identify independently?
➤ What types of cues were required to reach an adequate level of performance?
➤ How many hours does the patient have available in a day? In a week? Throughout the month?
➤ Did the patient complete a **Time Available Equation** on a regular basis? What types of cues were required for this performance?

Phase 5: Routines

Establishing routines can be an important aspect of time management. Many routine, daily tasks are difficult for patients with executive function deficits because they over- or under-attend to them. Patients frequently neglect daily tasks because they can't fit them into the day, or conversely, they spend too much time and attention on routine tasks for fear of forgetting them. Establishing a routine time for each task can insure its completion.

Discuss with the patient which aspects of daily life can be fairly routine and scheduled as such. If a patient describes never having time to leave and pick up clothes from the dry cleaner, consider whether this can be scheduled every Friday at 5:30.

Refer to the **Time Estimation Worksheet** and **Time Available Equation** to help the patient determine what activities occur regularly. Here are some typical routines:
➤ waking up
➤ performing morning routine
➤ performing evening routine
➤ grocery shopping
➤ doing laundry
➤ taking clothes to dry cleaners
➤ doing errands
➤ housecleaning
➤ maintaining car

Work with the patient to assign these tasks to specific, routine times, taking appropriate consideration to the time needed for each. Have the patient enter these routines into his or her monthly and daily calendar.

Helpful Hints: Just because the phone is ringing does not mean it must be answered. View the phone as a tool to assist, not control. If the patient reports getting off task at work or home because he or she becomes distracted by the phone, schedule a time to take and receive calls and rely on voice mail for the others. Establish a schedule for checking voice mail messages and returning calls every day at routine times.

Some patients describe becoming distracted by the E-mail alarm when working online. Have the patient learn how to disengage the visual and auditory alarm feature during work periods. Schedule a routine time to check and answer E-mail.

Touch mail only once and act on it immediately: file it, refer it to someone else, or throw it out.

Sunday	Monday	Tuesday	Wednesday	Thursday	Friday	Saturday
1 Do Wash	**2**	**3** 9:00 Meet with Bob 12:00 Lunch 6:00 Meeting	**4** Get Gasoline	**5** Lauren Birthday Grocery Shop	**6** Clothes to Cleaners	**7**
8 Do Wash	**9** Pick up Clothes	**10**	**11** 10:00 DDS	**12** Grocery Shop	**13**	**14** James Birthday
15 Do Wash	**16** 12:00 Jan Lunch	**17** Mom & Dad Anniversary	**18** Get Gasoline	**19** Grocery Shop	**20** Clothes to Cleaners	**21**
22 Do Wash	**23** Pick up Clothes	**24**	**25**	**26** Grocery Shop	**27** Pay Day	**28** 8:00 Party
29 Do Wash	**30** Holiday 2:30 Picnic	**31**				

	OCTOBER 3
6:00	Wake and Shower
7:00	Eat Breakfast
7:30	Leave for Work
8:00	Planning **Check Voice Mail** **Check E-mail**
8:30	Meet with Bob
9:00	**Morning Phone Calls**
10:00	**Check Voice Mail**
10:15	
11:00	
11:30	Drive to Lunch **Check Voice Mail**

12:00	Lunch at Main Street **Get Gasoline**
1:00	Drive Back from Lunch
1:30	**Check E-mail** **Afternoon Phone Calls**
2:00	**Check Voice Mail**
2:15	
3:00	
4:00	**Check E-Mail**
4:15	
5:00	Organize for Tomorrow **Check Voice Mail**
5:30	Drive to Meeting
6:00	Meeting at Club
7:00	Drive Home
7:30	Dinner

Documentation:
➤ What percentage of routines were written into the schedule on a regular basis?
➤ How many of these were completed as scheduled, rescheduled, or abandoned?
➤ What prevented the patient from completing a routine task at the routine time? Was there a pattern to the errors?

Phase 6: To-Do Lists

To-do lists can prove to be an invaluable aspect to the patient's time organization. During the morning schedule review, the patient should determine what tasks need to be completed during the day. This must be comprehensive and include all required

Helpful Hint: Break the habit of writing on numerous "sticky notes." The to-do list needs to be in the organizational system, not on a separate sheet of paper.

daily events, including tasks at home and at work, as well as social activities. Some actions on the list must be done at a specific time and should be scheduled to reflect that time commitment. Others may be more loose and can be listed along the side or at the bottom.

To Do List:	
Errands:	❑ Drop off clothes at dry cleaners ❑ Go to drugstore
Work:	❑ Finish project and turn in
Misc.	❑ Meeting at club tonight

	OCTOBER 3
6:00	Wake and Shower
7:00	Eat Breakfast
7:30	Leave for Work
8:00	**Bring Clothes for Dry Cleaners to Work** Planning Check Voice Mail Check E-mail
8:30	Meet with Bob
9:00	Morning Phone Calls
10:00	**Confirm Meeting Tonight** Check Voice Mail
10:15	
11:00	
11:30	Drive to Lunch Check Voice Mail
12:00	Lunch at Main Street Get Gasoline
1:00	Drive Back from Lunch
1:30	Check E-mail Afternoon Phone Calls
2:00	Check Voice Mail
2:15	
3:00	
4:00	Check E-Mail
4:15	
5:00	**Project Due** Organize for Tomorrow Check Voice Mail
5:30	Drive to Meeting
6:00	**Drop Off Clothes at Dry Cleaners** **Go to Drugstore** Meeting at Club
7:00	Drive Home
7:30	Dinner

Documentation:
➤ Did the patient create a daily to-do list?
➤ Was the list all-encompassing?
➤ In hindsight, how many items failed to make the list yet needed to be done?
➤ Were there particular items or categories that the patient always forgot?

Phase 7: Prioritizing

At this point, the patient has recorded all scheduled events in the organizational system, established a daily to-do list, and determined the time necessary to complete each event. Rarely, however, are the number of hours in the day compatible with the amount to be completed. Patients with executive function disorders tend to be haphazard in deciding which tasks to complete and which to let go. Patients with frontal lobe dysfunction have difficulty filtering what is and what is not a priority. Determination of priorities must be based on a structured priority system.

Have the patient establish the priorities for each day by considering a priority paradigm such as the following:

	Pressing	Not Pressing
Significant	Tasks which are both crucial to complete and have a deadline	Tasks which are crucial to complete but do not have a deadline
Not Significant	Tasks which may not be crucial but must be done within a time constraint	Tasks which are neither crucial nor under time constraints

Another way to consider priorities is to apply a penalty/bonus paradigm.

	High Bonus	Low Bonus
Penalty	Tasks that render benefit and involve punishment from others if not completed	Tasks that render little benefit and involve punishment from others if not completed
No Penalty/ Reward	Tasks that render benefit and reward from others when completed	Tasks that render little benefit but induce rewards from others when completed

Patients with difficulties in time management often work exclusively in the pressing/significant box or the penalty boxes. Due to their inability to effectively manage their time, they do not deal with a task until it becomes driven by a deadline or a crisis. Because they are always operating in these boxes, they rarely find time for events that are not pressing or significant.

Ask the patient to identify the most important item on his or her to-do list for each day and physically mark it with **#1** on the daily calendar. This is an item that must be completed that day. Next, have the patient identify the **#2** item, a task which would be nice to complete but is not necessary, and mark that on the calendar.

Helpful Hint:	Too many priorities, by definition, are not priorities. There should never be more than 2-3 #1 items in a day.

To-Do List:	
Errands:	☐ Drop off clothes at dry cleaners ☐ Go to drugstore
Work:	☐ Finish project and turn in
Misc.	☐ Meeting at club tonight

	OCTOBER 3
6:00	Wake and Shower
7:00	Eat Breakfast
7:30	Leave for Work
8:00	Bring Clothes for Dry Cleaners to Work Planning Check Voice Mail Check E-mail
8:30	**#1** Meet with Bob
9:00	Morning Phone Calls
10:00	Confirm Meeting Tonight Check Voice Mail
10:15	
11:00	
11:30	Drive to Lunch Check Voice Mail
12:00	Lunch at Main Street Get Gasoline
1:00	Drive Back from Lunch
1:30	Check E-mail Afternoon Phone Calls
2:00	Check Voice Mail
2:15	
3:00	
4:00	Check E-Mail
4:15	
5:00	**#1** Project Due Organize for Tomorrow Check Voice Mail
5:30	Drive to Meeting
6:00	Drop Off Clothes at Dry Cleaners **#2** Go to Drugstore Meeting at Club
7:00	Drive Home
7:30	Dinner

Documentation:

➤ Did the patient establish an appropriate number of priorities for the day?

➤ Did he or she use a paradigm to determine the priority, carefully considering all aspects?

➤ Into which box do most of the tasks fall?

➤ Were the items established as #1 priority consistently being completed?

Phase 8: Review Times Three

Writing down the information is only half of the equation. Looking at what was written down is the other half. The patient should review and study the time schedule at least three times per day.

The first opportunity is in the morning when the patient plans the day. Review will occur again midday, with the purpose of examining the events that have occurred and anticipating the remaining activities.

 Helpful Hint: Correlating review times with meal times is an effective way to target 3 review periods in the day.

Lastly, the schedule will be reviewed in the evening to both recall the current day's events and to look toward the following day.

Write a large *1*, *2*, and *3* on each day's page that correspond to a morning (1), mid-day (2), and evening (3) review of the day's events. Require the patient to cross off the number to each review as it is accomplished. If the patient has significant difficulty remembering to check the organizational system, attach a small clip-on alarm that is set to go off at determined times.

1   **2**   **3**

	OCTOBER 3
6:00	Wake and Shower
7:00	Eat Breakfast
7:30	Leave for Work
8:00	Bring Clothes for Dry Cleaners to Work Planning **+ Review Period #1** Check Voice Mail Check E-mail
8:30	#1 Meet with Bob
9:00	Morning Phone Calls
10:00	Confirm Meeting Tonight Check Voice Mail
10:15	
11:00	
11:30	Drive to Lunch Check Voice Mail **Review Period #2**
12:00	Lunch at Main Street Get Gasoline
1:00	Drive Back from Lunch
1:30	Check E-mail Afternoon Phone Calls
2:00	Check Voice Mail
2:15	
3:00	
4:00	Check E-Mail
4:15	
5:00	#1 Project Due Organize for Tomorrow **+ Review Period #3** Check Voice Mail
5:30	Drive to Meeting
6:00	Drop Off Clothes at Dry Cleaners #2 Go to Drugstore Meeting at Club
7:00	Drive Home
7:30	Dinner

Documentation:
- ➤ How frequently did the patient review the schedule? Three times per day?
- ➤ What percentage was the patient averaging during this treatment period?
- ➤ What kept the patient from being successful in checking the calendar?
- ➤ Was there a pattern to the missed reviews?

Phase 9: Feed Forward

Even if the patient is appropriately scheduling his or her day within the time constraints and with appropriate priorities, there will still be some items that are not accomplished. Where do these items go? Individuals with executive function disorders often abandon tasks if they are not completed at the time they were scheduled. At the end of each day, the patient should review the schedule for tasks that were not completed. Each incomplete task should be evaluated as follows:

Opportunity Missed:	The event was a one-time opportunity. By not doing it, the chance was missed and the event is over.
Feed Forward:	The scheduled item could be done at another time. Immediately schedule this event forward in the calendar system.
Store for Later:	The item remains interesting but a definitive time to complete it is not necessary. Log this in the **Master List** (see Phase 12 on page 70) for future reference.

Documentation:
- ➤ How many items were not completed?
- ➤ Were they priorities?
- ➤ Of the items on the daily to-do list that were not completed, how many were appropriately dealt with in terms of rescheduling or entering elsewhere?

1　　　　　　　　　**2**　　　　　　　　　**3**

OCTOBER 3	
6:00	Wake and Shower
7:00	Eat Breakfast
7:30	Leave for Work
8:00	Bring Clothes for Dry Cleaners to Work Planning + Review Period #1 Check Voice Mail Check E-mail
8:30	#1 Meet with Bob
9:00	Morning Phone Calls
10:00	Confirm Meeting Tonight Check Voice Mail
10:15	
11:00	
11:30	Drive to Lunch Check Voice Mail Review Period #2
12:00	Lunch at Main Street Get Gasoline
1:00	Drive Back from Lunch
1:30	Check E-mail Afternoon Phone Calls
2:00	Check Voice Mail
2:15	
3:00	
4:00	Check E-Mail
4:15	
5:00	#1 Project Due Organize for Tomorrow + Review Period #3 Check Voice Mail
5:30	Drive to Meeting
6:00	Drop Off Clothes at Dry Cleaners (**Missed — Move to Friday**) #2 Go to Drugstore Meeting at Club (**Missed — Attend Next Month**)
7:00	Drive Home
7:30	Dinner

Phase 10: Anticipation

Once mastery of a single day of scheduled events is complete, the patient should move toward anticipation of more than one day. Patients with executive function disorders are often working minute to minute, just trying to keep their heads above water. They have no time or forethought to consider a report due on Friday until Thursday.

In this phase of therapy, patients need to anticipate full weeks of schedules at a time. Consider the number and type of appointments for each day, the amount of time needed to complete projects, and the amount of time available. A patient may need to have snacks for her son's 30 classmates for Thursday but have a full day of activities scheduled for Wednesday. The only opportunity to shop is on Tuesday morning. The patient with frontal lobe dysfunction isn't able to recognize this dilemma until Wednesday night when she checks the next day's schedule. Assist the patient in learning how to start at the end date/deadline for the project and work back to determine when the project fits in.

Documentation:
➤ Can the patient develop weekly schedules and weekly to-do lists?
➤ How many activities during the week did the patient feel he or she had to deal with abruptly?

1   **2**   **3**

	OCTOBER 3
6:00	Wake and Shower
7:00	Eat Breakfast
7:30	Leave for Work
8:00	Bring Clothes for Dry Cleaners to Work Planning + Review Period #1 Check Voice Mail Check E-mail
8:30	#1 Meet with Bob
9:00	Morning Phone Calls
10:00	Confirm Meeting Tonight Check Voice Mail
10:15	
11:00	
11:30	Drive to Lunch Check Voice Mail Review Period #2
12:00	Lunch at Main Street Get Gasoline
1:00	Drive Back from Lunch
1:30	Check E-mail Afternoon Phone Calls **Collect Information for Report Due Next Monday**
2:00	Check Voice Mail
2:15	
3:00	
4:00	Check E-Mail
4:15	
5:00	#1 Project Due Organize for Tomorrow + Review Period #3 Check Voice Mail
5:30	Drive to Meeting
6:00	Drop Off Clothes at Dry Cleaners (Missed — Move to Friday) **Take Suit for Tuesday Meeting** #2 Go to Drugstore Meeting at Club (Missed — Attend Next Month)
7:00	Drive Home
7:30	Dinner

Phase 11: Expect the Unexpected

"The best laid plans . . . ." Wonderfully modeled time schedules rarely go as planned. A schedule can be altered for so many reasons and it is impossible to anticipate all situations. It is, however, possible to anticipate some. In looking at the daily schedule, the patient should ask, "What could possibly go wrong?" Planning ahead is highly problematic for the patient with executive function disorders, and the repair phase is discussed in more detail in other sections of this book (see page 155). For treatment purposes, take a given day in the patient's schedule and contrive an unexpected change. Have the patient describe the possible solutions and schedule necessary changes.

For example, at 3:00 the patient's schedule reads, "Pick up kids at school and drive to piano lessons." Suggest an unexpected situation such as, "When you go outside, the car tire is flat." Then ask, "How does this impact the rest of the schedule and how will you reschedule?"

Documentation:
- ➤ How flexible was the patient in both contrived and actual schedule changes?
- ➤ How completely did the patient deal with the items in conflict?
- ➤ How many tasks did the patient forget when a schedule change occurred?

Phase 12: The Master List

One dilemma, not unique to executive function disorders, is balancing short-term to long-term tasks and goals. Short-term activities, those that can be completed within a week, should be listed on daily to-do lists. However, most of us have activities we would like to accomplish, yet they do not fit into a specific time frame. These ideas should go onto a "master list." This is a single, continuous, dynamic list that provides the patient with a place to "keep things in mind." It is not intended as an action list, so there is no need to limit the items on this list or to categorize them. The list may be long, and it may stay that way. Instruct the patient to frequently re-examine the list, eliminate items that are no longer interesting or necessary, add items as they come up, and group similar items.

During weekly planning, have the patient review the master list. Is there an opportunity to fit one of these items into the week?

Master List

Work:
- ❏ Investigate new tax program.
- ❏ Develop new review form.
- ❏ Take course in technology.
- ❏ Rearrange office space.

Home:
- ❏ Look for new couch.
- ❏ Purchase new bookshelf.
- ❏ Organize closet.
- ❏ Have dinner with the Smiths.

Documentation:
- ➤ Did the patient add items to the master list on an ongoing basis?
- ➤ Were there items on the daily to-do list that would be more appropriate for the master list and vice versa?
- ➤ How frequently did the patient review the master list?

Sticking to a rigid time schedule may be difficult for some patients whose style is more carefree. If the patient is consistently missing appointments or deadlines, has difficulty scheduling daily tasks, complains of constantly being behind or hurried, or is generally disorganized, a time schedule is essential. It is easy to back off of some of the rigidity as the patient proves ability.

Time Estimation Worksheet

Name:	Date:

Make a list of various tasks you need to accomplish (getting dressed, making phone calls, driving to appointments, shopping, etc.). Estimate the amount of time you think it will take to complete each task. After you have completed a task, write the actual amount of time you spent doing it.

Task	Estimate	Actual

Time Available Equation

Name:	Date:

Time Available

Write daily tasks on the lines below and the amount of time (in hours) tasks take in the shaded boxes. Continue subtracting from the subtotals to calculate the time available every day outside of normal tasks and routines.

hours in a (circle one)   **day**   **work week**

_____

subtotal

_____

subtotal

_____

subtotal

_____

subtotal

_____

Total Hours Available

Attention

Deficits in attention are common following frontal lobe damage. For the purpose of this manual, we will consider five components of attention:

➤ **Focused Attention** is the ability to respond discretely to particular visual, auditory or tactile stimuli.

➤ **Sustained Attention** is the ability to sustain a steady response during continuous activity. It incorporates the notion of vigilance and concentration.

➤ **Selective Attention** is the ability to maintain attention in the face of distracting or competing stimuli. These distractions may be either external or internal.

➤ **Alternating Attention** is the capacity for mental flexibility that allows the shift of focus between tasks.

➤ **Divided Attention** is the ability to respond simultaneously to multiple tasks or to do more than one activity at a time.

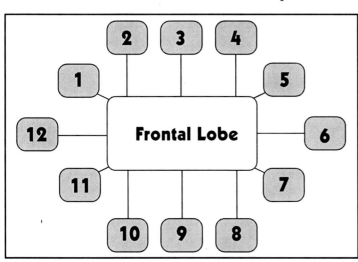

Picture attention as an electrical fuse box. Lots of current travels in and out without difficulty; however, once the electrical circuit approaches maximum capacity, it does not take much for it to "blow." Whether the input is from switching on a small light or a huge microwave may not matter . . . too much is too much. And once the circuits blow, it takes time to reset everything and get back to normal. The key is to instruct patients to operate below maximum and avoid having the circuits blow.

Copyright © 2003 LinguiSystems, Inc.

With normal function, the frontal lobe will organize/store the details of jobs 1-4 and 6-12 while it focuses on job 5. It can set down job 5 and pick up job 8 and focus on it, and so on. It can add job 13 or 14, or when finished with job 5, plug in a new job 5.

The injured frontal lobe can't organize or separate the details of jobs 1-12. Each seems of equal importance at all times. If the person tries to focus on job 5, every other job vies for equal time and attention. There is so much input it is impossible to focus. If the frontal lobe is on overload, it cannot absorb anything else. It shuts down and refuses to accept any more input and nothing gets done.

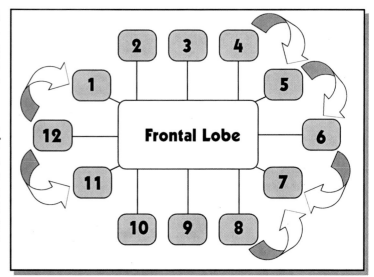

The frontal lobe can deal magnificently with one job at a time, on a linear level, seeing each job to its completion before adding another job.

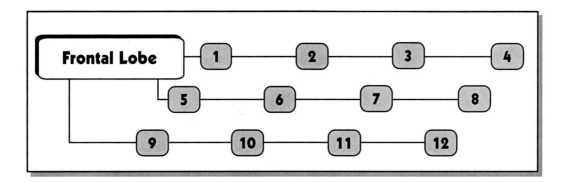

In order to be successful in the remediation and/or the compensations for attention deficits, the patient needs to be knowledgeable about the types of attention.

➤ Begin by instructing the patient in definitions and examples of each type of attention.

➤ As the patient is learning types of attention, have him or her discern what type of attention is required to successfully complete a variety of daily tasks.

Copyright © 2003 LinguiSystems, Inc.

Task	Required attention levels
Reading the paper	Sustained
Reading the paper with the radio on	Sustained + Selective
Reading the paper with the radio on and listening for the weather report	Sustained + Divided
Reading the paper with the radio on and listening to a breaking new story	Sustained + Alternating
Talking on the phone	Sustained
Talking on the phone with others in the room	Sustained + Selective
Talking on the phone with others asking you questions	Sustained + Alternating
Talking on the phone while preparing a can of soup	Sustained + Divided

Have patients use the **Required Attention Levels** chart on page 98 to keep track of tasks and types of attention levels over several days. If the patient works outside of the home, he or she should complete the chart for work activities also. Ask the patient to identify which activities were particularly difficult and which were simple. In analyzing this chart, the patient will become more aware of the attentional demands of the activities participated in daily. This knowledge can change "I can't do it!" to "I have trouble concentrating for long periods of time." By recognizing the specific demands of the activity, employing appropriate strategies to maximize abilities becomes more obvious.

As with all treatment tasks, the more functional and "everyday" the activity the better. Use specific drill activities only as supplements to daily activities.

Focused Attention

This level of attention is a lower-level ability of discrimination and not typically impaired with higher-level disorders such as executive function disorders.

Sustained Attention

Sustained attention is the ability to maintain attention to the task for a long enough period of time to complete the task. Throughout the day, a person needs adequate sustained attention to read the paper, drive a car, or complete a phone conversation.

There are several variables to consider in maintaining attention to a task.

➤ **Difficulty of the task:** It is far more difficult to sustain attention to a difficult activity as compared to a more simplistic activity. Complexity can be of either a physical or mental nature.

➤ **Familiarity:** It is generally more difficult to sustain attention to an activity that is novel; however, extremely familiar tasks may become mundane and therefore challenging to sustained attention.

➤ **Enjoyment:** It is easier to maintain attention to a task that is fun to do as compared to one that is not enjoyable.

It is important to have a realistic understanding of how long a task can engage attention. Even a simple, familiar, enjoyable activity can only capture attention for approximately 20 minutes before a small break is needed. Often, 15-30 seconds can be enough of a pause before returning to the task. Difficulty arises when persisting at a task long after attention has waned and/or taking too long to return to the task after a break.

The most effective strategy to compensate for reduced sustained attention is to predetermine the length of concentration time on a task and the length and fashion of the break. Attention should be controlled, not controlling.

Target activities that the patient participates in frequently—simple and complex, familiar and novel, enjoyable and boring. Guide the patient through completing the **Activity Worksheet** on page 99 to identify the activity, predetermine the concentration period, the break period, and the break activity.

Next, have the patient actually participate in these activities while timing/regulating the concentration time and break time. Upon completion, identify if this particular equation was successful and what alterations should be made. Ask the patient to continue with this activity until success is frequent.

An example of a completed **Activity Worksheet** is shown on the next page.

Activity	Concentration Time	Break Time & Activity	Was It Successful? Why?	Modifications
Reading the newspaper	3 paragraphs	*30 seconds* Look up from the paper and review the main point.	Yes	Increase to 5 paragraphs.
Reading a book	5 minutes	*30 seconds* Look up from the book and review the plot of the story.	No; didn't recall details of the last 2 paragraphs.	Decrease time to 4 minutes.
Listening to a lecture	20 minutes	*30 seconds* Look up, put down pen, take a sip of water, and count to 30.	Yes	Continue; do not increase.
Watching a movie at home	30 minutes	*30 seconds* Pause movie, get up, and stretch.	No; didn't follow the plot of the movie.	Decrease watching time to 20 minutes.
Cleaning the house	30 minutes	*5 minutes* Stop, sit down, and have a drink.	No; started watching TV during break and didn't return to cleaning.	Keep TV off and set timer/ alarm for 5 minutes during break.
Paying bills	15 minutes	*1 minute* Get up and walk around the desk.	No; became distracted and didn't return to bills for 30 minutes.	Use alarm or timer to remind when break is over.

➤ Begin this chart during treatment sessions with the patient identifying a real-life activity and the therapist determining the times and break activities.

➤ Move toward the patient developing the entire chart during sessions using treatment tasks.

➤ Lastly, move toward having the patient use this chart at home, and then review the findings during treatment.

Helpful Hint: Completing even long, complicated tasks is possible when they are broken down into small, manageable increments. Kitchen timers are inexpensive, easily-available tools to signal break and return times.

In addition to managing reduced sustained attention via compensations, patients can work on both clinical and functional tasks to increase the length of time they are able to attend. Highly structured, systematic increases of the amount of time a patient persists with a task can be successful in increasing the overall time period a patient is able to attend to an action. Real-life activities are best to use. Have the patient practice reading, paying bills, typing, or writing during the treatment session and homework for the pure activity of practice. Systematically increase the attention times. Several clinical tasks for improving sustained attention are described on the following pages.

➤ **Cancellation Tasks:** These simple tasks provide excellent clinical tasks for attention. The **Cancellation Activities** on pages 100-115 consist of a number of visual cancellation tasks that use shapes, numbers, letters, etc.

Introducing the Task:
- "Here is a page of arrows pointing in various directions. Make a slash through each arrow that is pointing *up*. I'll ask you to stop in about 1 minute."

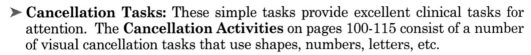

Manipulating the Difficulty of the Task:
- Manipulate the length of time the task is continued.
- Manipulate the frequency with which the target appears.
- Manipulate the visual difficulty of the task (e.g., print size).

➤ **Math Equations:** For those who enjoy math, a page of simple math equations such as those on pages 116-121 can be used for sustained attention tasks.

- Have the patient perform the equations for specified amounts of time. Here are some examples of simple math equations included in the activities:

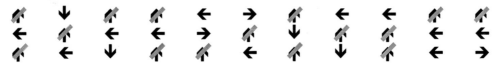

$$\begin{array}{cccccccc} 1 & 2 & 4 & 4 & 3 & 1 & 6 & 7 \\ +9 & +7 & +2 & +6 & +2 & +7 & +5 & +7 \\ \hline 10 & 9 & 6 & 10 & 5 & 8 & 11 & 14 \end{array}$$

Introducing the Task:
- "Here is a page of single-digit addition problems. I'd like you to solve them. I'll tell you to stop in about 1 minute."
- "Here is a page of single-digit addition problems. I'd like you to solve them. I'll tell you to stop in about 5 minutes."
- Here is a page of 3-digit addition problems. I'd like you to solve them. I'll tell you to stop in about 1 minute."

Manipulating the Difficulty of the Task:
- Manipulate the length of time the patient persists with the task.
- Manipulate the difficulty of the math problems.
- Manipulate the visual stimulation of the page, (e.g., print size).

➤ **Auditory Attention:** In these tasks, the patient listens as you read a list of random words, names, or numbers aloud. Have the patient make a tally mark whenever he or she hears the target word, name, or number. Use the **Auditory Attention** activities on pages 122-132 for this task.

Introducing the Task:
- "Here is a blank sheet of paper. I am going to read a random list of names at a fast pace. Every time you hear the name *Mary* I want you to make a tally mark. You will do this for about 1 minute."

Mary	Joan	**Mary**	Fred	Alice	Bob	Susan
Betty	**Mary**	Lauren	Martha	**Mary**	Sally	George

- "Here is a blank sheet of paper. I am going to read a random list of numbers. I would like you to make a tally mark every time you hear a number containing a *7*. You will do this for about 2 minutes."

121	**367**	481	**167**	652	841	925	**763**	**467**	208
325	**947**	881	621	**371**	444	**973**	602	**187**	134

Manipulating the Difficulty of the Task:
- Manipulate the length of time the patient persists with the task.
- Manipulate the speed of presentation.
- Manipulate the complexity of the stimuli.
- Manipulate the complexity of the target:
  - ✔ "Make a mark every time you hear a number that ends in *7*."
  - ✔ "Make a mark every time you hear a number that is greater than *3*."
  - ✔ "Make a mark every time you hear a word that begins with a *T*."
  - ✔ "Make a mark every time you hear a word that begins with a vowel."

Selective Attention

Selective attention is the ability to concentrate on the target task while ignoring distractions. At a basic level, it requires selecting one stimulus to pay attention to from a group or a series, like finding certain letters in a word search or listening for a specific highway during a traffic report. At a higher level, it is trying to follow a conversation and to ignore another conversation taking place nearby. Distractions may be external (TV or radio) or internal (hunger). During the day, counting change in a loud grocery store, talking on the phone with family members talking in the same room, or participating in a meeting following only 2 hours sleep the night before are all examples of selective attention.

There are several variables to consider in keeping attention focused on the target while ignoring the distractions:

➤ **Difficulty of the task:** Although at first thought, a simple target task would appear easiest, tasks that are too simple or mindless are often the easiest to drift from.

➤ **Familiarity:** It is easier to attend to a familiar task. Conversely, it is more difficult to tune out a familiar task in lieu of concentrating on the less familiar target activity.

➤ **Enjoyment:** It is easier to tune out distractions when the target task is pleasurable. Conversely, it is more difficult to tune out a distraction that is preferable to the target task.

➤ **Intensity of the distraction:** The amount of effort needed to tune out a distraction often leaves little left for the target task.

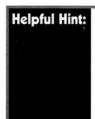 **Helpful Hint:** Silence is not always golden. For many, a completely silent environment greatly increases internal distractions. Activity or noise in the background can become white noise and actually enhance some patients' ability to attend to the task at hand.

The obvious compensation for reductions in selective attention is to reduce the distractions. To do this, the patient must become keenly aware of what is occurring concurrently with the target task.

Begin by asking the patient to complete the **Distractions Worksheet** on page 133 during the treatment session using real-life scenarios. An example of a completed chart is on the next page.

Task	Distractions Present	Modifications
Driving to work	• Radio on • Talking on phone • Busy highway • Hot • Hungry	• Turn off radio. • Limit phone calls. • Consider an alternate route. • Take off coat. • Eat breakfast.
Writing a letter	• Phone ringing • Radio on news station • Poor quality pen • Thinking of another letter that needs to be written	• Turn on voice mail. • Change to quiet music. • Have all supplies before writing letter. • Schedule a time to write second letter; keep note card handy for ideas.
Making dinner	• TV on • Talking on phone • Children asking questions about homework • Stove and microwave both active • Hungry	• Turn off TV or mute the volume. • Make calls before or after preparation time. • Schedule time before or after dinner for homework help. • Use timers to keep varied finish times on track. • Have a small snack.
Attending a meeting	• Noisy air conditioner • Thinking about new ideas stimulated from discussion • Sleepy	• Select a seat far away from blower. • Keep note cards handy to make memos to self. • Sip on water; change meeting time.

➤ Begin this chart during treatment sessions with the patient identifying a real-life activity and the therapist determining the distractions and modifications.
➤ Move toward the patient developing the entire chart during sessions.
➤ Lastly, move toward having the patient use this chart at home and then review the findings during treatment.

Ultimately, the patient must become aware of the distractions that may be preventing completion of the task at hand and become aware of appropriate modifications to both the target task and the competing tasks, allowing for success.

In addition to managing reduced sustained attention via compensations, patients can work on both clinical and functional tasks to increase their ability to tolerate distractions.

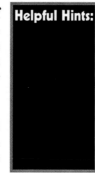

Helpful Hints:

• Have the patient use a sign on the door or on the desk at work to communicate to people when not to disturb him or her.

• Remember, attention is cumulative. Do not forget to incorporate the patient's limits of sustained attention into his or her plans for selective attention.

Highly structured, systematic increases of the amount and intensity of distractions can be successful. Have the patient perform reading, paying bills, typing, writing or other functional tasks during the treatment session and for homework for the pure activity of practice. Systematically manipulate these variables:
- difficulty of the task
- familiarity of the task
- enjoyment of the target task
- enjoyment of the distraction
- intensity of the distraction

For example, turn on a news radio channel or a TV news channel. Ask the patient to listen carefully to a story and write down a few facts about the story. As the patient is listening, read aloud a competing story from the newspaper. Here are some ways to further manipulate the difficulty of this task:
- Manipulate the interest level of the target story.
- Manipulate the interest level of the competing story.
- Manipulate the proximity/intensity of the target story.
- Manipulate the proximity/intensity of the competing story.

As with all treatment, the more "true to life" the treatment activity, the easier the generalization to the patient's life. That said, there is benefit to nonfunctional, clinical tasks; however, they should never be used in exclusion.

➤ **Cancellation Tasks:** The **Cancellation Activities** on pages 100-115 provide excellent clinical tasks for selective attention. Select a target letter, number, or shape and have the patient scan the page and mark off the target every time it appears while there is a simultaneous distraction, such as a radio or TV playing in the background.

Manipulating the Difficulty of the Task:
- Manipulate the variables described in the **Sustained Attention** section (length of time the task is continued, frequency with which the target appears, visual difficulty of the task).
- Manipulate the intensity of the distracting stimuli.
- Manipulate the interest level of the distracting stimuli.
- Manipulate the number of distractions.

You can also use everyday reading materials, such as newspapers and magazines, to present a cancellation task. Here are some ways to introduce that type of activity incorporating various types and intensities of distractions:
- "Here is the newspaper. I'd like you to cross off the letter *t* every time it appears in this article. While you are doing this, I'll have some quiet music on in the background. Ignore the music and work on the letters. You'll do this for about 1 minute."
- "Here is the newspaper. I'd like you to cross off the letter *t* every time it appears in this article. I'm going to have on some loud rock music in the background. Ignore the music and work on the letters. You'll do this for about 1 minute."
- "Here is the newspaper. I'd like you to cross off the letter *t* every time it appears in this article. We're going to do this in the cafeteria, and I'm going to be talking with someone next to you. Ignore these distractions and concentrate on the letters. You'll do this for about 1 minute."

➤ **Math Equations:** For those who enjoy math, a page of simple math equations, such as the ones on pages 116-121, can be used for selective attention tasks. Have the patient perform the equations for specified amounts of time in the presence of competing stimuli, such as a conversation in the background.

Manipulating the Difficulty of the Task:
- Manipulate the length of time the patient persists with the task.
- Manipulate the difficulty of the math problems.
- Manipulate the visual stimulation of the page (e.g., print size).
- Manipulate the intensity of the distraction.
- Manipulate the interest of the distraction.
- Manipulate the number of distractions.

 Copyright © 2003 LinguiSystems, Inc.

➤ **Auditory Selective Attention:** The **Auditory Attention** activities on pages 122-132 provide excellent clinical tasks for selective attention. These simple tasks can be easily manipulated to address attention issues. Read a list of random names or numbers aloud to the patient. Have the patient make a tally mark whenever the target letter is read.

Introducing the Task:
- "Here is a blank sheet of paper. I am going to read a random list of words. I would like you to make a tally mark every time you hear the word *for*. At the same time, I will have some soft music on in the background. Concentrate on my voice and ignore the music. You will do this for about 1 minute."
- "Here is a blank sheet of paper. I am going to read a random list of names at a fast pace. I'm also going to have the radio playing on the news station. Every time you hear the name *Bob,* I want you to make a tally mark. Ignore the radio and concentrate on my voice. You will do this for about 1 minute."
- "Here is a blank sheet of paper. I am going to read a random list of numbers. I would like you to make a tally mark every time you hear a number containing a *7*. We're going to sit in a corner in the waiting room to do this. Ignore the people and voices and concentrate on my voice. You will do this for about 2 minutes."

Have the patient perform the task for specified amounts of time and vary the task by reading aloud words, numbers, or names.

Manipulating the Difficulty of the Task:
- Manipulate the length of time the patient persists with the task.
- Manipulate the speed of presentation.
- Manipulate the intensity of the competing stimuli.
- Manipulate the interest level of the competing stimuli.
- Manipulate the complexity of the target.
  - ✔ "Make a mark every time you hear a number that ends in *7*."
  - ✔ "Make a mark every time you hear a number that is greater than *3*."
  - ✔ "Make a mark every time you hear a word that begins with a *T*."
  - ✔ "Make a mark every time you hear a word that begins with a vowel."

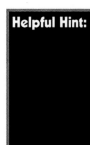

Helpful Hint: Most speech-language pathology offices provide ideal conditions. The room is quiet, well-lit, and temperature-controlled. Taking treatment outside the office is a quick way to manipulate the level of distraction. Try having the treatment session in the waiting room, physical therapy gym, or even the local coffee house.

Copyright © 2003 LinguiSystems, Inc.

➤ **Visual Selective Attention:** Ask the patient to read aloud a page of words with visual foils, such as the ones presented on pages 133-137. For example, the words *big* and *little* appear in both large and small print. Ask the patient to read the word, ignoring the size of the print. Conversely, ask the patient to state the size of the print, inhibiting the desire to read the word. Activities are also provided to do similar activities with the words *skinny/fat, cursive/print,* and *bold/light.*

Introducing the Task:
- "Look at the words on this page. Scan word by word, saying *big* for every word printed in all capital letters and *little* for all words printed in lowercase."

BIG	LITTLE	big	little	LITTLE	big
BIG	LITTLE	big	LITTLE	big	little
little	big	BIG	LITTLE	big	BIG

Answer:

big	big	little	little	big	little
big	big	little	big	little	little
little	little	big	big	little	big

Alternating Attention

The ability to fluctuate attention between two or more activities is called *alternating attention.* This skill is utilized frequently in daily activities, such as making dinner, stopping to answer the door, then returning to cooking; balancing the checkbook, stopping to put new batteries in the calculator, and then returning to the checkbook; or listening to a business meeting, stopping to answer a phone call, then returning to the meeting.

There are several variables of difficulty that contribute to alternating attention abilities.
- ➤ **Difficulty of each task:** It is easier to alternate between simple tasks.
- ➤ **Familiarity of each task:** It is easier to alternate between known tasks.
- ➤ **Enjoyment:** It is easier to alternate between enjoyable tasks.
- ➤ **Number of tasks alternating between:** The more tasks involved, the more difficult.
- ➤ **Length of time allowed working on each task:** There is a critical point on both ends of the time spectrum. Spending too much time on one task makes it easy to forget to return to the other(s). Spending too little time on each task makes things confusing.

 Copyright © 2003 LinguiSystems, Inc.

➤ **Length of time between tasks:** Again, there is a critical point at both ends. Spending too much time between tasks results in a loss of sustained attention. Spending too little time between tasks becomes confusing.

➤ **Length of time to persist with these tasks:** It is much easier to alternate between two simple, fun tasks for a few minutes than for an hour.

To assist patients in becoming aware of the number of tasks they function between, ask them to complete the **Task Combination Worksheet** on page 138. Here is an example of a completed worksheet:

Tasks	Appropriate Combinations	Times	Reminders
Do laundry Cook dinner	Do laundry + cook dinner.	10 minutes to start wash. Begin dinner for 30 minutes ➔ change laundry for 10 minutes. Return to dinner for 30 minutes ➔ change laundry for 10 minutes.	Use kitchen timer. Use pencil to mark your place in the recipe. Use kitchen timer. Use pencil to mark your place in the recipe.
Help with homework	Homework help cannot be combined with others.		

➤ Ask the patient to generate a list of activities for the day. These will include daily and routinely scheduled tasks, along with particular activities for that day.

➤ Work with the patient to determine which of these tasks need to be completed in isolation and which can be alternated between.

➤ Considering the difficulty, familiarity, and enjoyment of each task, predetermine the number of tasks that can be involved, the length of time the patient will spend on each task, the time between tasks, and the total time this alternating will continue.

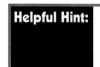 **Helpful Hint:** Remember that attention is cumulative. Do not forget to incorporate the patient's limits of sustained and selective attention into the plan.

➤ Additionally, determine a reminder method to trigger when to end one task and begin the next. This may be an alarm clock, timer, watch alarm, phone call, etc.

In addition to managing reductions in alternating attention via compensations, patients can work on both clinical and functional tasks to increase their ability to alternate between tasks. Highly structured, systematic increases of the amount, difficulty, and time constraints of tasks can be successful. Have the patient perform a variety of activities during the treatment session and homework for the pure activity of practice.

Systematically manipulate these variables:
- **Difficulty of each task:** It is easier to alternate between simple, routine tasks.
- **Familiarity of each task:** It is easier to alternate between familiar tasks.
- **Enjoyment:** It is easier to alternate between pleasant tasks.
- **Number of tasks attention is divided between:** Fewer tasks are easier.
- **Length of time the patient must persist with each task:** Too little time with each task is confusing, but too much time can result in ignoring the additional tasks.
- **Length of time allowed between tasks:** Again, too little transition time can become confusing, but too much transition time can result in failing to begin or return to the other task.

➤ **Cancellation Tasks:** The **Cancellation Activities** on pages 100-115 provide excellent clinical tasks for alternating attention. These simple tasks can be easily manipulated to address various attention issues.

Introducing the Task:
- Have the patient cross off the same target for 5 lines (up arrow). At the 6th line ask the patient to cross off a different target for the next 5 lines (down arrow). At the 10th line have the patient return to the original target, etc.

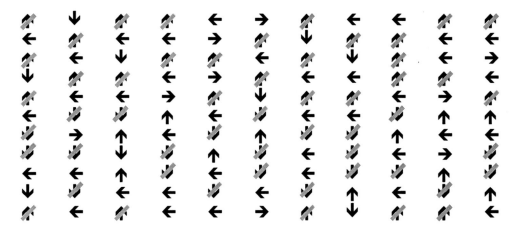

Manipulating the Task:
- Manipulate the variables as described in the Sustained Attention section.
- Manipulate how frequently the patient is required to switch targets. For example, instead of switching targets every 5 lines, have the patient change every 3 lines, and eventually switching every line.
- Manipulate the pattern or predictability of changing to a different target. For example, during the scanning task, randomly say "switch," at which time the patient must switch to a different target.

- Manipulate how many target stimuli the patient is alternating between. For example, he or she may begin by scanning for 1 target (crossing off only the "up" arrows) and progress to scanning for 3 targets (crossing off the "up," "down," and "left" arrows).

➤ **Math Equations:** For those who enjoy math, a page of simple math equations such as those on pages 139-141 can be used for alternating attention tasks. Alternating the function of the math equation is one way to get the patient to alternate attention.

Manipulating the Task:
- Manipulate the variables described in the **Sustained Attention** section.
- Manipulate how frequently the patient is required to switch targets. For example, the activity on page 139 provides the patient with alternating lines of addition and subtraction problems.
- Manipulate the pattern or predictability of changing to a different target. For example, the activity on page 140 presents lines of mixed addition and subtraction problems.
- Manipulate how many functions the patient is required to alternate between. For example, the activity on page 141 presents lines of mixed addition, subtraction, and multiplication problems.

The key to improving high-level alternating attention is to *systematically* increase the variables regardless of the clinical or functional tasks patients are engaged in doing.
- Begin with two simple, enjoyable tasks. Provide adequate time to "get into" each task, for example 3-5 minutes. Provide a 30-second break between tasks. Continue with these two tasks for 2-3 cycles.
- Increase the difficulty relative to the patient's area of trouble. For example, maintain all the parameters in the previous step, but increase the number of tasks to be alternated between to 3.

Vs.

Continue with 2 tasks but make the tasks themselves more difficult.

Vs.

Continue with 2 tasks but decrease the amount of time allowed on each task to 1 minute.

Vs.

Decrease the amount of time between tasks to 5 seconds.

Vs.

Continue the tasks for 4-5 cycles.

- Ultimately you will increase all these parameters such that the patient would be required to do multiple, difficult tasks for 30 seconds each, with no break in between for 15-20 minutes.

Here are some ways to systematically increase variables in a cancellation task:

- "I'm going to give you a page filled with symbols. I would like you to cross off the *heart* every time you see it for these first 5 lines. For the next 5 lines I would like you to cross off the *diamond*. Continue to alternate back and forth between hearts and diamonds every 5 lines."

- "I'm going to give you a page filled with symbols. I would like you to cross off the *heart* every time you see it for these first 3 lines. For the next 3 lines I would like you to cross off the *diamond*. Continue to alternate back and forth between hearts and diamonds every 3 lines."

- "I'm going to give you a page filled with symbols. I would like you to cross off the *heart* every time you see it on this first line. For the next line I would like you to cross off the *diamond*. Continue to alternate back and forth between hearts and diamonds every line."

- "I'm going to give you a page filled with symbols. I would like you to begin by crossing off all the *hearts* you see. In about 15 seconds I will say *diamond* and for the next time period you should cross off the diamonds. Continue to alternate back and forth between hearts and diamonds every time I instruct you to switch."

➤ **Agitating Alternating**

To work on alternating between various tasks, set up different "stations" that the patient will alternate between. Here are some suggestions for the stations:

- Manipulate colored blocks. Provide the patient with 10 "blueprints" stating the order or position where the blocks should be placed.
- Write the alphabet omitting the letters in your name.
- Read a newspaper article.
- Do a computer activity.
- Balance a checkbook.
- Solve simple puzzles.
- Alphabetize lists of words/papers.
- Set an alarm clock.
- Write the alphabet backwards.
- Count backwards from 100 by 4 (written or oral).
- Count forward by 5, then subtract 3 (written or oral).
- Do simple pegboard tasks.
- Perform simple reasoning activities.
- Complete an application.
- Write a letter of complaint.
- Write or copy a paragraph intentionally failing to dot all *i*'s and cross all *t*'s.

Divided Attention

The ability to do more than one thing at a time is **divided attention**. Dividing attention occurs often in daily life, such as when someone is driving, cooking, or working. The difficulty arises in determining how many tasks can attention successfully be divided among.

There are several variables of difficulty that contribute to divided attention skills.

➤ **Difficulty of each task:** It is easier to divide attention between simple tasks.

➤ **Familiarity of each task:** It is easier to divide attention between known tasks.

➤ **Enjoyment:** It is easier to divide attention between enjoyable tasks.

➤ **Number of tasks attention is divided between:** The more tasks involved, the more difficult.

➤ **Length of time you must persist with these tasks:** It is easier to divide attention for shorter periods of time.

To assist patients in becoming aware of the number of tasks they function between, ask them to complete the **Simultaneous Tasks Worksheet** on page 142 (a completed chart from the worksheet is on the next page). Having the patient complete the chart during a treatment session will be difficult, since it requires the person to recall the number of functions he or she attempted at one time. Therefore, this is an activity that a patient frequently needs to complete as homework and review during the session.

Divided attention tasks can easily be simplified by switching them to alternating attention tasks. For example, instead of making the coffee and the toast at the same time, make the coffee and then make the toast.

Helpful Hint: Both alternating attention and divided attention fall under the heading of "multi-tasking." Today's society values the ability to "multi-task," which is essentially the ability to alternate or divide attention. The data is beginning to show, however, that multi-tasking is not saving any time, in fact it may be taking longer to complete tasks and they may be less accurate than if they are done one at a time. Helping the patient to be sharply aware of his or her abilities and limitations with alternating and divided attention will ultimately assist the patient in being successful in completing tasks, whether they are done one at a time or simultaneously.

Simultaneous Tasks	Problems	Modifications
Listening to weather Taking a shower	None	None
Making coffee Making toast Reading the paper Listening to the news	Lost track of number of coffee scoops Burned the toast	Prepare water and coffee grounds the evening before. Don't read the paper until seated and breakfast is done.
Driving to work Listening to voice mail	Forgot message	Listen to voice mail at home or at work.
Working on the computer Making phone calls Interruptions from co-workers	Lost data while on phone Failed to complete project	Turn on voice mail while working. Put a sign on your door requesting no interruptions.
Reading Watching favorite TV show	Missed the main point of both the book and the TV show	Tape show or defer reading until after the show is over.

In addition to managing reductions in divided attention via compensations, patients can work on both clinical and functional tasks to increase their ability to divide attention between tasks. Highly structured, systematic increases of the amount and difficulty of tasks can be successful. Have the patient perform a variety of activities during the treatment session and homework for the pure activity of practice. Systematically manipulate the following variables:

- the difficulty of each task
- the familiarity of each task
- the enjoyment of each task
- the number of tasks between which the patient is dividing attention

➤ **Cancellation Tasks:** The **Cancellation Activities** presented on pages 100-115 provide excellent clinical tasks for alternating attention. These simple tasks can be easily manipulated to address various attention issues.

Introducing the Task:

- "Here is a page of random letters. I want you to cross out the letter *t* and the letter *z* every time they appear. You'll do this for about 1 minute."

Helpful Hint: An excellent and readily available tool for cancellation tasks is the daily newspaper, which can be used for targeting different letters or numbers in different frequencies.

- "Here is a page of random letters. I want you to cross out the letter *t* every time it appears. I will be reading you a short news story. I want you to listen to the story while working on the letters, and I'll ask you some questions about it when we are done. You will do this for about 1 minute."

- "Here is a page of random letters. I want you to cross out the letter *t* and the letter *a* every time they appear. While you are doing this I want you to listen to this weather forecast and be able to tell me the temperature tomorrow. You'll do this for about 3 minutes."

Manipulating the Task:

- Have the patient scan for more than 1 target at a time.
- Manipulate the variables as described in the **Sustained Attention** section.
- Manipulate the variables as described in the **Selective Attention** section; however, require the patient to pay attention to the distracting stimuli. For example, have the patient continue crossing out letters while listening to a news story and stating the main point.
- Manipulate the variables as described in the **Alternating Attention** section.
- Manipulate the number of target items scanned for.

Copyright © 2003 LinguiSystems, Inc.

➤ **Math Equations:** For those who enjoy math, a page of simple math equations (pages 116-121 and 139-141) can be used for divided attention tasks. Require the patient to complete math problems while attending to other tasks simultaneously. For example, have the patient solve the math problem while listening to a news story or carrying on a conversation.

Manipulating the Task:
- Manipulate the variables as described in the **Sustained Attention** section.
- Manipulate the variables as described in the **Selective Attention** section; however, require the patient to attend to the distracting stimuli. For example, have the patient continue to cross out the designated target(s) while listening to a news story and stating the main point of the story.
- Manipulate the variables as described in the **Alternating Attention** section.
- Manipulate the number of target items scanned for.

➤ **Odd/Even Tasks:** Ask the patient to sort a grid of numbers by odds/evens in either ascending or descending order using the activities on pages 143-145.

Introducing the Task:
- "Here is a grid of numbers. I want you to sort the numbers by writing all the even numbers on the right side of the page and the odd numbers on the left. Put the smallest number at the top and then sort the numbers smallest to largest."

Manipulating the Task:
- Increase the amount of numbers on the grid.
- Increase the complexity of the numbers.

For any given task within the patient's schedule, ask him or her to identify the stipulations of attention:
- For how long is the patient required to sustain attention? Is that amount of time within the patient's ability? Is there a way to reduce the time prior to the patient failing at the task?
- Will there be competing stimuli? Is there a way to decrease or eliminate that competition before encountering it?
- Will the patient be asked to do more than one thing at a time? Is that within the patient's ability? Is there a way to reduce the alternating and divided attention constraints prior to the activity?

➤ **Mental Flexibility:** Mental flexibility is the ability to see familiar situations in a different fashion, handle different situations in different ways, and to respond effectively to new situations. It involves the ability to do these things:
- see things from several different perspectives
- adapt to change
- learn from mistakes
- solve problems in new ways

When mental flexibility is impaired, patients perform well in familiar situations when everything goes as planned, but in new situations, or old situations with surprises, they exhibit difficulties. Faced with something unfamiliar, patients either overlook its newness and treat it as a version of something familiar, or they recognize its newness and treat it as difficult.

In order to alternate or divide attention, or participate successfully in the repair phase (discussed in the next chapter, beginning on page 155), patients must possess the ability to be flexible in their thinking. The ability to mentally go down one path, stop, go down another path, stop, and so forth, is a skill that is often impaired with executive function disorders.

Analyze situations from the patient's life experiences asking questions such as:
- Was there another way you could have done the activity?
- Was there another choice?
- How many solutions did you consider before trying this one?
- Did this go as originally planned? What alterations did you make if it didn't?

Direct practice in mental flexibility can be helpful. The **Homonyms Activities** on pages 146-149 are a linguistic task in mental flexibility. Present the words on those pages to your patients and see how many different meanings he or she can determine for the target word. Here are some examples:

- ***bowl***   a dish for eating cereal
         to play a sport with a ball and pins
         an important college football game

- ***spring***   a season of the year
         a coil
         to jump up suddenly
         a small stream or brook

The **Trail Activities** on pages 150-153 provide another task to promote mental flexibility. Give the patient a copy of one of the pages containing letters of the alphabet and numbers. Ask the patient to connect the letters and numbers in order but in an alternating fashion, for example, A-1-B-2-C-3 etc., as in the example pictured here.

Mental flexibility can also be practiced by playing a rule-shifting card game. Sort a deck of playing cards, and have the patient work to determine why a card is included in the "Yes" pile as opposed to the "No" pile based upon predetermined criteria known only to the therapist. For example, if the predetermined rule is "only red cards":

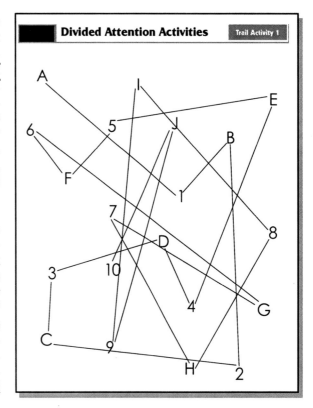

Divided Attention Activities   Trail Activity 1

- The patient turns over the 3 of hearts and the therapist says "Yes."
- The patient turns over the 4 of spades, the therapist says "No."

Once the patient has ascertained the rule, the therapist switches to another rule, without notification. For example, this time the predetermined rule is "only even numbers":

- The patient turns over the 3 of diamonds and the therapist says "No."
- The patient turns over the 8 of clubs and the therapist says "Yes."

See the **Rule Shift List** on page 154 for suggestions of predetermined rules.

Required Attention Levels

| Name: | Date: |

Task	Required Attention Levels
1.	
2.	
3.	
4.	
5.	
6.	
7.	
8.	
9.	
10.	
11.	
12.	
13.	
14.	
15.	

Activity Worksheet

Name: _____ | Date: _____

Activity	Concentration Time	Break Time & Activity	Was It Successful? Why?	Modifications

f p o i a u t o i b n o k j

p o t u o i t j a o v j p i

u j v o i j i u o y j l k m

l k s d j o i t u r e o s i

j s k v k n b u i y e u k j

h z i y t z y f i u s g m f

n l k p o t k l m l y p o y

k m l k m k f d j g i h s g

k j b v j s a f u y a b v d

k g h i u t r k j o i j n o

p j o i b i h u i c g y u q

y y u g h i o v w j m o i n

j o r i o y k p o p e i o w

u i w e h r u q t r a b k j

n b m n l g k u p o m n m o

i t s u g i n m n v k u a y

i u y f i u h f n k v n n v

m z b v h u z g f u z g f y

t q g y u e h t i h s y j d

o j m l k n m l m n p b j n

d i o j g h o i u h f a u y

```
i  j  n  o  o  i  b  i  h  u  i  c  g
y  u  q  y  y  u  g  h  i  o  v  w  j
o  r  i  o  y  k  p  o  p  e  i  o  w
u  i  w  e  h  r  u  q  w  t  r  a  b
k  j  n  b  m  n  l  g  k  u  p  g  n
m  n  v  k  u  a  y  i  u  y  f  i  u
h  f  n  k  v  n  n  v  m  z  b  v  h
u  z  g  f  u  z  g  f  y  t  q  g  y
u  e  h  t  i  h  s  y  j  d  o  j  m
l  k  n  m  l  m  n  p  b  j  n  d  i
q  j  g  h  o  i  u  h  f  a  u  y  w
f  i  b  v  k  j  g  n  v  l  k  s  m
h  j  h  p  o  i  e  r  j  h  k  m  b
o  i  s  p  j  g  o  i  h  g  a  i  u
h  u  i  w  n  c  q  n  v  y  u  i  a
f  u  y  a  b  v  d  k  g  h  i  u  t
r  k  j  o  i  j  n  o  p  j  o  i  b
i  h  u  i  c  g  y  u  q  y  u  u  g
h  i  o  v  w  j  m  o  i  n  e  o  r
i  o  y  k  p  o  p  e  i  o  w  b  h
r  u  q  w  t  r  a  b  o  w  b  i  m
n  l  g  k  u  p  o  m  k  j  i  y  t
s  u  g  i  n  m  n  v  n  m  o  n  i
u  y  f  i  u  h  f  n  k  v  a  n  v
m  z  b  v  h  u  z  g  f  u  z  g  f
y  t  q  g  y  u  e  h  t  i  h  s  y
j  d  o  j  m  l  k  n  u  i  w  n  c
q  n  v  y  u  i  a  f  u  f  p  o  i
a  u  t  o  i  b  n  o  k  u  p  o  t
u  o  i  t  j  a  o  v  j  p  i  u  j
v  o  i  j  i  u  o  g  j  l  k  u  l
k  s  d  j  o  i  t  u  r  e  o  s  i
j  s  k  v  k  n  b  u  i  y  e  u  k
j  h  z  i  y  t  z  y  f  i  u  s  g
m  f  n  l  k  p  o  t  k  l  m  l  y
p  o  y  k  m  l  k  m  k  f  d  j  g
i  h  s  g  k  j  b  v  j  s  a  r  u
y  a  b  v  d  k  g  h  i  u  t  i  k
j  o  i  j  n  o  p  j  o  i  b  r  h
u  i  c  g  y  u  q  y  y  u  g  h  i
o  v  w  j  m  o  i  n  j  o  r  i  o
```

```
i j n o o i b i h u i c g z y u q y y u g h i o v
w j o r i o y k p o p e i o w u i w e h r u q w t
a b q k j n b m n l g k u p g n o m n v k u a y i
y f i u y h f n k v n n v m z b v h v u z g f u z
f y t q g y u u e h t i h s y j d o j m t l k n m
m n p b j n d i a q j g h o i u h f a u y w a f i
v k j g n v l k s m o h j h p o i e r j h k m b y
i s p j g o i h g a i u g h u i w n c q n v y u i
v f u y a b v d k g h i u t n r k j o i j n o p j
i b w i h u i c g y u q y y u g s h i o v w j m o
n j o r q i o y k p o p e i o w e h t r u q w t r
b k j n b m r n l g k u p o m n m o i t v s u g i
m n v k u a y i x u y f i u h f n k v n n v w m z
v h u z g f u z g f y y t q g y u e h t i h s y a
d o j m l k n u i w n c b q n v y u i a f u f p o
c a u t o i b n o k j p o t e u o i t j a o v j p
u j d v o i j i u o g j l k m l f k s d j o i t u
e o s i h j s k v k n b u i y e u k g j h z i y t
y f i u s g i m f n l k p o t k l m l y j p o y k
l k m k f d j g k i h s g k j b v j s a f u l y a
v d k g h i u t r k m j o i j n o p j o i b i h n
i c g y u q y y u g h i p o v w j m o i n j o r i
y k p o p e i f p o i a u t o i b n o k j p o t u o
t j a o v j p i u j v o i j i j l k m l k s d j o
i t u r e o s i j s k v k n a u i y e u k j h z i
y t z y f i u s g m f n l k p c t k l m l y p o y
k m l k m k f d j g i h s g k j u v j s a f u y a
b v d k g h i u t r k j o i j n o w j o i b i h u
i c g y u q y y u g h i o v w j m o x n j o r i o
y k p o p e i o w u i w e h r u q t r z b k j n b
m n l g k u p o m n m o i t s u g i n m a v k u a
y i u y f i u h f n k v n n v m z b v h u b g f u
z g f y t q g y u e h t i h s y j d o j m l d n m
l m n p b j n d i o j g h o i u h f a u y w f e b
v k j g n v l k s m h j h p o i e r j h k m b o f
s p j g o i h g a i u h u i w n c q n v y u i a f
y a q v d k g h i u t r k j o i j n o p j o i b i
u i c g y u q y y u g h i o v w j m o i n j o r i
y k p o p o w u i w e h r u q w t r a b k j n b m
l g k u p o m t r k m j o i j n o p j o i b i h n
i c g y u q y y u g h i p o v w j m o i n j o r i
y k p o p e i f p o i a u t o i b n o k j p o t u o
t j a o v j p i u j v o i j i j l k m l k s d j o
i t u r e o s i j s k v k n a u i y e u k j h z i
b v d k g h i u t r k j o i j n o w j o i b i h u
```

F P O I A U T O I B N O K J

P O T U O I T J A O V J P I

U J V O I J I U O Y J L K M

L K S D J O I T U R E O S I

J S K V K N B U I Y E U K J

H Z I Y T Z Y F I U S G M F

N L K P O T K L M L Y P O Y

K M L K M K F D J G I H S G

K J B V J S A F U Y A B V D

K G H I U T R K J O I J N O

P J O I B I H U I C G Y U Q

Y Y U G H I O V W J M O I N

J O R I O Y K P O P E I O W

U I W E H R U Q T R A B K J

N B M N L G K U P O M N M O

I T S U G I N M N V K U A Y

I U Y F I U H F N K V N N V

M Z B V H U Z G F U Z G F Y

T Q G Y U E H T I H S Y J D

O J M L K N M L M N P B J N

D I O J G H O I U H F A U Y

I	J	N	O	O	I	B	I	H	U	I	C	G
Y	U	Q	Y	Y	U	G	H	I	O	V	W	J
O	R	I	O	Y	K	P	O	P	E	I	O	J
U	I	W	E	H	R	U	Q	W	T	R	A	B
K	J	N	B	M	N	L	G	K	U	P	I	N
M	N	V	K	U	A	Y	I	U	Y	F	I	U
H	F	N	K	V	N	N	V	M	Z	B	V	H
U	Z	G	F	U	Z	G	F	Y	T	Q	G	Y
U	E	H	T	I	H	S	Y	J	D	O	J	M
L	K	N	M	L	M	N	P	B	J	N	D	I
Q	J	G	H	O	I	U	H	F	A	U	Y	W
F	I	B	V	K	J	G	N	V	L	K	S	M
H	J	H	P	O	I	E	R	J	H	K	M	B
O	I	S	P	J	G	O	I	H	G	A	I	U
H	U	I	W	N	C	Q	N	V	Y	U	I	A
F	U	Y	A	B	V	D	K	G	H	I	U	T
R	K	J	O	I	J	N	O	Q	J	O	I	B
I	H	U	I	C	G	Y	E	I	N	Y	O	G
H	I	O	V	W	J	M	O	I	O	J	E	R
I	O	Y	K	P	O	P	E	K	J	W	B	H
R	U	Q	W	T	P	A	B	N	O	N	I	M
N	L	G	K	U	P	O	M	K	M	O	Y	T
S	U	G	I	N	M	N	V	K	U	A	N	I
U	Y	F	V	H	H	F	N	F	U	N	G	V
M	Z	B	G	U	U	Z	G	T	I	Z	S	F
Y	T	Q	J	Y	U	E	H	U	H	H	N	Y
J	D	O	Y	M	L	K	N	U	I	W	O	C
Q	N	V	O	U	I	A	F	U	F	P	O	I
A	U	T	T	I	B	N	O	K	U	P	O	T
U	O	I	J	I	A	O	V	J	P	I	U	J
V	O	I	J	J	U	O	G	J	P	K	M	L
K	S	D	J	I	I	T	U	R	L	O	S	I
J	S	K	V	O	N	B	U	I	E	E	U	K
J	H	Z	I	K	T	Z	Y	F	Y	U	L	G
M	F	N	L	Y	P	O	T	K	I	M	J	Y
P	O	Y	K	M	L	K	M	K	L	D	J	G
I	H	S	G	K	J	B	V	J	F	A	F	U
Y	A	B	V	D	K	G	H	I	S	T	R	K
J	O	I	J	N	O	P	J	O	U	I	H	H
U	I	C	G	Y	U	Q	Y	J	I	G	I	I
O	V	W	J	M	O	I	N	J	O	R	I	O

```
U J D V O I J I U O G J L K M L F K S D J O I T U
E O S I H J S K V K N B U I Y E U K G J H Z I Y T
Y F I U S G I M F N L K P O T K L M L Y J P O Y K
L K M K F D J G K I H S G K J B V J S A F U L Y A
V D K G H I U T R K M J O I J N O P J O I B I H N
I C G Y U Q Y Y U G H I P O V W J M O I N J O R I
Y K P O P E I F P O I A U T O I B N O K J P O T U O
T J A O V J P I U J V O I J I J L K M L K S D J O
I T U R E O S I J S K V K N A U I Y E U K J H Z I
Y T Z Y F I U S G M F N L K P C T K L M L Y P O Y
K M L K M K F D J G I H S G K J U V J S A F U Y A
B V D K G H I U T R K J O I J N O W J O I B I H U
I C G Y U Q Y Y U G H I O V W J M O X N J O R I O
I J N O O I B I H U I C G Z Y U Q Y Y U G H I O V
W J O R I O Y K P O P E I O W U I W E H R U Q W T
A B Q K J N B M N L G K U P G N O M N V K U A Y I
Y F I U Y H F N K V N N V M Z B V H V U Z G F U Z
F Y T Q G Y U U E H T I H S Y J D O J M T L K N M
M N P B J N D I A Q J G H O I U H F A U Y W A F I
V K J G N V L K S M O H J H P O I E R J H K M B Y
I S P J G O I H G A I U G H U I W N C Q N V Y U I
V F U Y A B V D K G H I U T N R K J O I J N O P J
I B W I H U I C G Y U Q Y Y U G S H I O V W J M O
N J O R Q I O Y K P O P E I O W E H T R U Q W T R
B K J N B M R N L G K U P O M N M O I T V S U G I
M N V K U A Y I X U Y F I U H F N K V N N V W M Z
V H U Z G F U Z G F Y Y T Q G Y U E H T I H S Y A
D O J M L K N U I W N C B Q N V Y U I A F U F P O
C A U T O I B N O K J P O T E U O I T J A O V J P
Y K P O P E I O W U I W E H R U Q T R Z B K J N B
M N L G K U P O M N M O I T S U G I N M A V K U A
Y I U Y F I U H F N K V N N V M Z B V H U B G F U
Z G F Y T Q G Y U E H T I H S Y J D O J M L D N M
L M N P B J N D I O J G H O I U H F A U Y W F E B
V K J G N V L K S M H J H P O I E R J H K M B O F
S P J G O I H G A I U H U I W N C Q N V Y U I A F
Y A Q V D K G H I U T R K J O I J N O P J O I B I
U I C G Y U Q Y Y U G H I O V W J M O I N J O R I
Y K P O P O W U I W E H R U Q W T R A B K J N B M
L G K U P O M T R K M J O I J N O P J O I B I H N
I C G Y U Q Y Y U G H I P O V W J M O I N J O R I
Y K P O P E I F P O I A U T O I B N O K J P O T U O
T J A O V J P I U J V O I J I J L K M L K S D J O
I T U R E O S I J S K V K N A U I Y E U K J H Z I
B V D K G H I U T R K J O I J N O W J O I B I H U
```

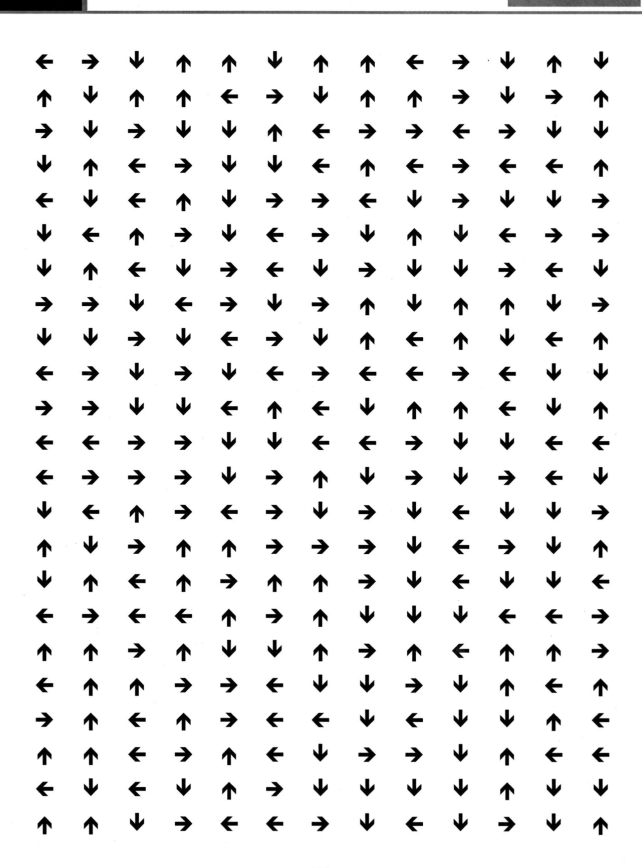

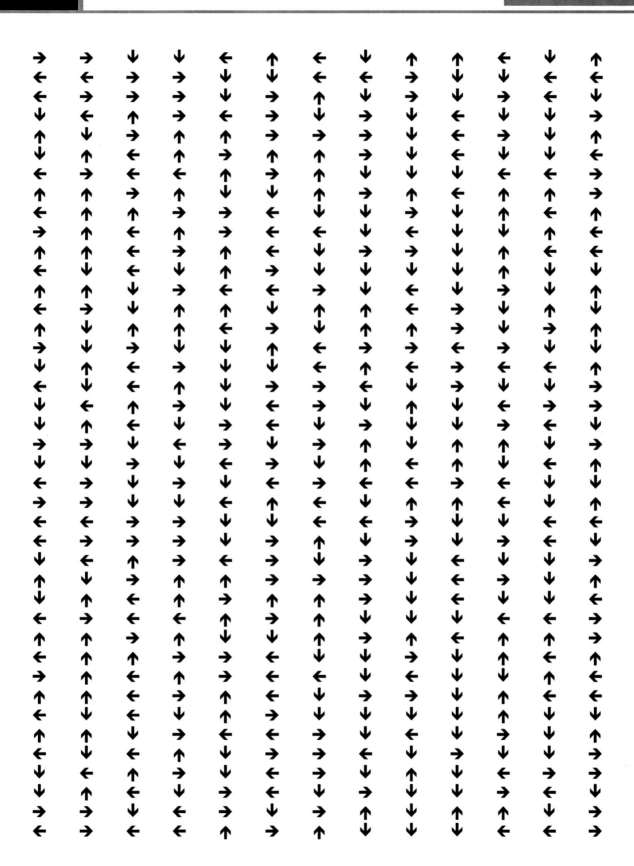

Cancellation Activities

☺	☹	😐	☺	☺	☹	☺	☺	😐	☹	☹	☺	☹
☺	☹	☺	☺	😐	😐	☹	☺	☺	☹	☹	☹	☺
😐	☹	☺	☹	☹	☺	😐	☹	😐	😐	☺	☹	☹
☹	☺	😐	☹	☹	☹	😐	☺	😐	😐	😐	😐	☺
😐	☹	😐	☺	☹	☺	☹	😐	☹	😐	☹	☹	☺
☹	😐	☺	☹	☹	😐	😐	☹	☺	☹	😐	☺	☹
☹	☺	😐	☹	😐	😐	☹	☺	☹	☹	☹	😐	☹
😐	☺	☹	😐	☹	☹	😐	☺	☹	☺	☺	☹	😐
☹	☹	☹	☹	😐	☺	☹	☺	😐	☺	☹	😐	☺
😐	☺	☹	☹	☹	😐	😐	😐	😐	☺	😐	☹	☹
☹	😐	☹	☹	😐	☺	😐	☹	☺	☺	😐	☹	☺
😐	😐	☺	☹	☹	☹	😐	😐	😐	☹	☹	😐	😐
😐	☺	☹	😐	☹	☺	☺	☹	☹	☹	😐	😐	☹
☹	😐	☺	☺	😐	☹	☹	😐	☹	😐	☹	☹	☺
☺	☹	☹	☺	☺	😐	☺	☹	☹	😐	😐	☹	☺
☹	☺	😐	☺	☺	☺	☺	☹	☹	😐	☹	☹	😐
😐	😐	😐	😐	☺	☺	☺	☹	☹	☹	😐	😐	☹
☺	☺	😐	☺	☹	☹	☺	☺	☺	😐	☺	☺	☹
😐	☺	☺	😐	☺	😐	☹	☹	☹	☹	☺	😐	☺
😐	☺	😐	☺	☺	😐	😐	☹	😐	☹	☹	☺	😐
☺	☺	😐	☹	☺	😐	☹	😐	☺	☹	☺	😐	😐
😐	☹	😐	☹	☺	☹	☹	☹	☹	☹	☺	☹	☹
☺	☺	☹	😐	😐	😐	☺	☹	😐	☹	☹	☹	☺

 Copyright © 2003 LinguiSystems, Inc.

Cancellation Activities

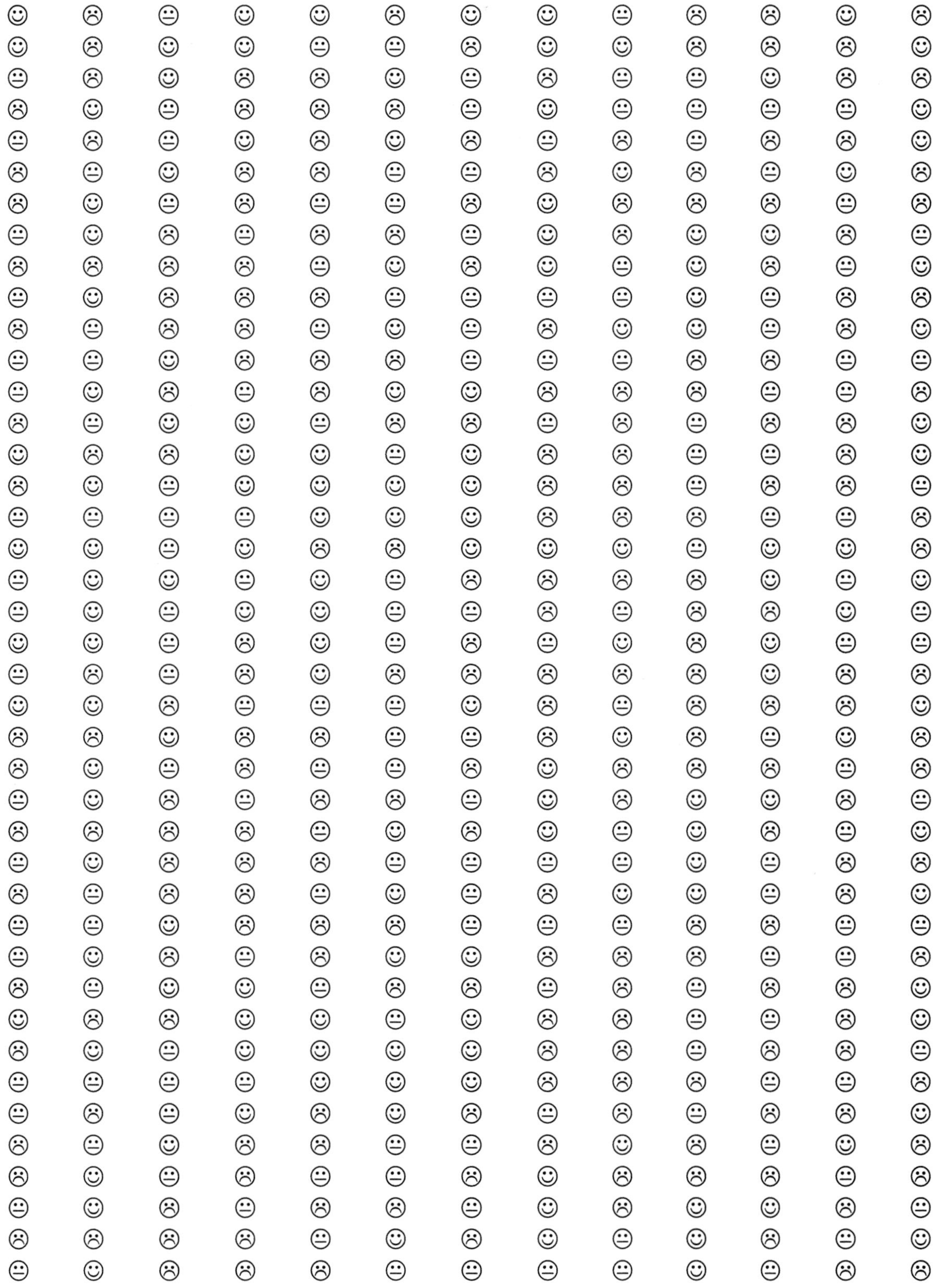

Copyright © 2003 LinguiSystems, Inc.

÷ + − ÷ ÷ + ÷ ÷ − + + ÷ +

÷ + ÷ ÷ − − + ÷ ÷ + + + ÷

− + ÷ + + ÷ − + − − ÷ + +

+ ÷ − + + + − ÷ − − − − ÷

− + − ÷ + ÷ + − + − + + ÷

+ − ÷ + + − − + ÷ + − ÷ +

+ ÷ − + − − + ÷ + + + − +

− ÷ + − + + + − ÷ + ÷ ÷ + −

+ + + + − ÷ + ÷ − ÷ + − ÷

− ÷ + + + − − − − ÷ − + +

+ − + + − ÷ − + ÷ ÷ − + ÷

− − ÷ + + + − − − + + − −

− ÷ + − + ÷ ÷ + + + − − +

+ − ÷ ÷ − + + − + − + + ÷

÷ + + ÷ ÷ − ÷ + + − − + ÷

+ ÷ − ÷ ÷ ÷ ÷ + + − + + −

− − − − ÷ ÷ ÷ + + + − − +

÷ ÷ − ÷ + + ÷ ÷ ÷ − ÷ ÷ +

− ÷ ÷ − ÷ − + + + + ÷ − ÷

− ÷ − ÷ ÷ − − + − + + ÷ −

÷ ÷ − + ÷ − + − ÷ + ÷ − −

− + − + ÷ + + + + + ÷ + +

÷ ÷ + − − − ÷ + − + + + ÷

```
+  ÷  −  +  +  ÷  +  +  −  ÷  ÷  +  ÷
+  ÷  +  +  −  −  ÷  +  +  ÷  ÷  ÷  +
−  ÷  +  ÷  ÷  +  −  ÷  −  −  +  ÷  ÷
÷  +  −  ÷  ÷  ÷  −  +  −  −  −  −  +
−  ÷  −  +  ÷  +  ÷  −  ÷  −  ÷  ÷  +
÷  −  +  ÷  ÷  −  −  ÷  +  ÷  −  +  ÷
÷  +  −  ÷  −  −  ÷  +  ÷  ÷  ÷  −  ÷
−  +  ÷  −  ÷  ÷  −  +  ÷  +  +  ÷  −
÷  ÷  ÷  ÷  −  +  ÷  +  −  +  ÷  −  +
−  +  ÷  ÷  ÷  −  −  −  −  +  −  ÷  ÷
÷  −  ÷  ÷  −  +  −  ÷  +  +  −  ÷  +
−  −  +  ÷  ÷  ÷  −  −  −  ÷  ÷  −  −
−  +  ÷  −  ÷  +  +  ÷  ÷  ÷  −  −  ÷
÷  −  +  +  −  ÷  ÷  −  ÷  −  ÷  ÷  +
+  ÷  ÷  +  +  −  +  ÷  ÷  −  −  ÷  +
÷  +  −  +  +  +  +  ÷  ÷  −  ÷  ÷  −
−  −  −  −  +  +  +  ÷  ÷  ÷  −  −  ÷
+  +  −  +  ÷  ÷  +  +  +  −  +  +  ÷
−  +  +  −  +  −  ÷  ÷  ÷  ÷  +  −  +
−  +  −  +  +  −  −  ÷  −  ÷  ÷  +  −
+  +  −  ÷  +  −  ÷  −  +  ÷  +  −  −
−  ÷  −  ÷  +  ÷  ÷  ÷  ÷  ÷  +  ÷  ÷
+  +  ÷  −  −  −  +  ÷  −  ÷  ÷  ÷  +
÷  ÷  +  ÷  ÷  −  ÷  +  ÷  ÷  −  +  ÷
÷  +  −  ÷  −  −  ÷  +  ÷  ÷  ÷  −  +
−  +  ÷  −  ÷  ÷  −  +  ÷  +  +  ÷  −
÷  ÷  ÷  ÷  −  +  ÷  +  −  +  ÷  −  +
−  +  ÷  ÷  ÷  −  −  −  −  +  −  ÷  ÷
÷  −  ÷  ÷  −  +  −  ÷  +  +  −  ÷  +
−  −  +  ÷  ÷  ÷  −  −  −  ÷  ÷  −  −
−  +  ÷  −  ÷  +  +  ÷  ÷  ÷  −  −  ÷
÷  −  +  +  +  −  ÷  ÷  −  ÷  −  ÷  ÷
+  ÷  ÷  +  +  −  +  ÷  ÷  −  −  ÷  +
÷  +  −  +  +  +  +  ÷  ÷  −  ÷  ÷  −
−  −  −  −  +  +  +  ÷  ÷  ÷  −  −  ÷
−  ÷  −  +  ÷  +  ÷  −  ÷  −  ÷  ÷  +
÷  −  +  ÷  ÷  −  −  ÷  +  ÷  −  +  ÷
÷  +  −  ÷  −  −  ÷  +  ÷  ÷  ÷  −  −
−  +  ÷  −  ÷  ÷  −  +  ÷  +  +  ÷  −
÷  ÷  ÷  ÷  −  +  ÷  +  −  +  ÷  −  +
−  +  ÷  ÷  ÷  −  −  −  −  +  −  ÷  ÷
```

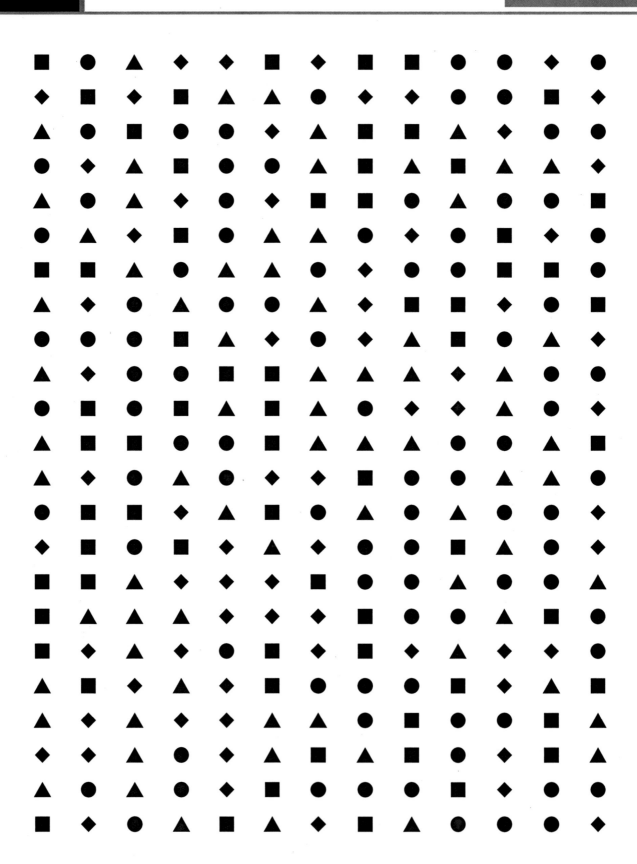

● ◆ ▲ ■ ● ● ▲ ■ ▲ ■ ▲ ▲ ◆
▲ ● ▲ ◆ ● ◆ ■ ■ ● ▲ ● ● ■
● ▲ ◆ ■ ● ▲ ▲ ● ◆ ● ■ ◆ ●
■ ■ ▲ ● ▲ ▲ ● ◆ ● ● ■ ■ ●
▲ ◆ ● ▲ ● ● ▲ ◆ ■ ■ ◆ ● ■
● ● ● ■ ▲ ◆ ● ◆ ▲ ■ ● ▲ ◆
▲ ◆ ● ● ■ ■ ▲ ▲ ▲ ◆ ▲ ● ●
● ■ ● ■ ▲ ■ ▲ ● ◆ ◆ ▲ ● ●
▲ ■ ■ ● ● ■ ▲ ▲ ▲ ● ● ▲ ■
▲ ◆ ● ▲ ● ◆ ◆ ■ ● ● ▲ ▲ ●
● ◆ ■ ◆ ▲ ■ ● ▲ ● ▲ ● ● ●
◆ ■ ● ■ ◆ ▲ ◆ ● ● ■ ▲ ● ◆
■ ■ ▲ ◆ ◆ ◆ ■ ● ● ▲ ● ● ▲
■ ▲ ▲ ▲ ◆ ◆ ◆ ■ ● ● ▲ ■ ●
■ ◆ ▲ ◆ ● ■ ◆ ■ ◆ ▲ ◆ ◆ ▲
▲ ■ ◆ ▲ ◆ ■ ● ● ● ■ ◆ ▲ ■
▲ ◆ ▲ ◆ ◆ ▲ ▲ ● ■ ● ● ■ ▲
◆ ◆ ▲ ● ◆ ▲ ■ ▲ ■ ● ◆ ■ ▲
▲ ● ▲ ● ◆ ■ ● ● ● ■ ◆ ● ●
■ ◆ ● ▲ ■ ▲ ◆ ■ ▲ ● ● ● ◆
◆ ▲ ● ● ■ ■ ▲ ▲ ▲ ◆ ▲ ● ●
● ■ ● ■ ▲ ■ ▲ ● ◆ ◆ ▲ ● ◆
▲ ■ ■ ● ● ■ ▲ ▲ ▲ ● ● ▲ ■
▲ ◆ ● ▲ ● ◆ ◆ ■ ● ● ▲ ▲ ●
● ■ ■ ◆ ▲ ■ ● ▲ ● ▲ ● ● ◆
◆ ■ ● ■ ◆ ▲ ◆ ● ● ■ ▲ ● ◆
■ ● ● ● ■ ■ ▲ ▲ ▲ ◆ ▲ ● ●
● ■ ● ■ ▲ ■ ▲ ● ◆ ◆ ▲ ● ◆
▲ ■ ■ ● ● ■ ▲ ▲ ▲ ● ● ▲ ■
▲ ◆ ● ▲ ● ◆ ◆ ■ ● ● ▲ ▲ ●
● ■ ■ ◆ ▲ ■ ● ▲ ● ▲ ● ● ◆
◆ ■ ● ■ ◆ ▲ ◆ ● ● ■ ▲ ● ◆
▲ ◆ ● ▲ ● ● ▲ ◆ ■ ■ ◆ ● ■

```
1   5   6   3   9   8   1   3   4   5   7   5   6
2   6   7   8   5   9   4   2   1   3   5   9   8
4   5   3   2   3   6   5   8   4   6   5   4   2
9   6   4   5   3   2   1   8   5   7   5   4   2
1   2   5   6   7   5   8   2   8   4   5   5   3
3   3   5   6   8   5   4   7   8   9   6   3   4
6   3   7   7   5   9   1   2   6   4   8   3   2
8   6   2   6   4   5   3   5   8   4   6   5   2
3   4   5   3   2   8   6   9   2   5   7   4   6
1   6   5   8   4   3   2   1   4   7   5   8   6
3   2   6   6   8   8   4   6   5   3   8   4   5
6   2   7   3   6   5   2   8   9   1   4   8   7
4   5   6   3   2   8   6   4   8   5   9   2   1
1   6   8   5   8   9   5   4   2   3   1   4   6
7   4   6   8   2   8   3   4   8   5   1   7   5
1   2   6   7   5   8   6   4   9   2   4   8   5
1   4   6   5   8   9   7   5   2   5   8   4   7
9   1   4   6   8   7   5   9   5   3   1   2   6
4   5   8   7   6   2   6   4   2   1   9   5   4
8   8   4   6   5   9   5   4   3   2   1   5   8
3   9   4   5   8   7   2   6   1   2   3   7   5
1   6   5   8   5   7   4   5   9   6   5   3   2
2   5   2   2   5   4   6   8   5   9   7   3   6
```

8	4	3	2	1	4	7	5	8	6	5	3	4
3	2	6	6	8	8	4	6	5	3	8	4	5
6	2	7	3	6	5	2	8	9	1	4	8	7
4	5	6	3	2	8	6	4	8	5	9	2	1
1	6	8	5	8	9	5	4	2	3	1	4	6
7	4	6	8	2	8	3	4	8	5	1	7	5
1	5	6	3	9	8	1	3	4	5	7	5	6
2	6	7	8	5	9	4	2	1	3	5	9	8
4	5	3	2	3	6	5	8	4	6	5	4	2
9	6	4	5	3	2	1	8	5	7	5	4	2
1	2	5	6	7	5	8	2	8	4	5	5	3
3	3	5	6	8	5	4	7	8	9	6	3	4
6	3	7	7	5	9	1	2	6	4	8	3	2
8	6	2	6	4	5	3	5	8	4	6	5	2
3	4	5	3	2	8	6	9	2	5	7	4	6
1	6	5	8	4	3	2	1	4	7	5	8	6
3	2	6	6	8	8	4	6	5	3	8	4	5
6	2	7	3	6	5	2	8	9	1	4	8	7
4	5	6	3	2	8	6	4	8	5	9	2	1
1	6	8	5	8	9	5	4	2	3	1	4	6
7	4	6	8	2	8	3	4	8	5	1	7	5
1	2	6	7	5	8	6	4	9	2	4	8	5
1	4	6	5	8	9	7	5	2	5	8	4	7
9	1	4	6	8	7	5	9	5	3	1	2	6
4	5	8	7	6	2	6	4	2	1	9	5	4
8	8	4	6	5	9	5	4	3	2	1	5	8
3	9	4	5	8	7	2	6	1	2	3	7	5
1	6	5	8	5	7	4	5	9	6	5	3	2
2	5	2	2	5	4	6	8	5	9	7	3	6
3	6	8	6	8	5	4	7	8	9	6	3	4
6	3	7	7	5	9	1	2	6	4	8	3	2
8	6	2	6	4	5	3	5	8	4	6	5	2
3	4	5	3	2	8	6	9	2	5	7	4	6
9	5	8	4	6	3	2	8	4	5	1	5	6
1	2	5	8	6	2	6	7	5	8	4	8	8
7	6	3	4	8	9	5	1	2	8	6	2	1

1 +9	2 +7	6 +5	4 +2	4 +6	3 +2	4 +6	1 +7	6 +5	7 +7	9 +2	8 +9	4 +7
5 +6	7 +9	5 +8	9 +2	1 +7	8 +6	5 +9	2 +4	8 +6	5 +8	6 +0	2 +9	7 +6
2 +9	0 +8	2 +5	7 +0	9 +9	8 +6	7 +0	1 +9	6 +2	8 +8	8 +6	7 +7	1 +5
9 +4	8 +9	3 +8	1 +1	5 +2	9 +7	8 +9	1 +8	7 +9	9 +5	0 +8	1 +0	7 +9
3 +9	2 +8	8 +1	6 +7	0 +2	9 +4	8 +7	6 +1	8 +9	9 +8	2 +4	7 +0	5 +1
9 +5	2 +9	5 +8	0 +7	9 +2	3 +9	8 +8	6 +5	0 +9	9 +8	2 +2	8 +5	2 +7
9 +5	8 +9	2 +0	5 +5	6 +4	0 +0	9 +7	3 +5	6 +0	0 +9	4 +6	9 +8	0 +3
9 +7	0 +4	8 +9	9 +8	8 +1	1 +0	7 +5	9 +9	8 +2	1 +0	4 +6	9 +9	1 +4
3 +9	6 +3	9 +5	5 +0	9 +2	7 +9	0 +9	5 +2	9 +0	7 +3	0 +8	5 +3	0 +9
0 +9	8 +1	5 +2	9 +4	0 +8	8 +1	2 +7	7 +4	9 +9	8 +0	2 +8	7 +7	8 +2
9 +0	8 +3	7 +8	9 +7	8 +0	6 +9	8 +6	4 +0	0 +3	9 +4	3 +9	8 +5	6 +9

Math Equations

9 −1	7 −2	6 −5	4 −2	6 −4	3 −2	6 −4	7 −1	6 −5	7 −7	9 −2	9 −8	7 −4
6 −5	9 −7	8 −5	9 −2	7 −1	8 −6	9 −5	4 −2	8 −6	8 −5	6 −0	9 −2	7 −6
9 −2	8 −0	5 −2	7 −0	9 −9	8 −6	7 −0	9 −1	6 −2	8 −8	8 −6	7 −7	5 −1
9 −4	9 −8	8 −3	1 −1	5 −2	9 −7	9 −8	8 −1	9 −7	9 −5	8 −0	1 −0	9 −7
9 −2	8 −2	8 −1	7 −6	2 −0	9 −4	8 −7	6 −1	9 −5	9 −8	4 −2	7 −0	5 −1
9 −5	9 −2	8 −5	7 −0	9 −2	9 −3	8 −8	6 −5	9 −0	8 −6	2 −2	8 −5	7 −2
9 −5	9 −8	2 −0	5 −5	6 −4	0 −0	9 −7	5 −3	6 −0	9 −0	6 −4	9 −8	3 −0
9 −7	4 −0	9 −0	9 −3	8 −1	1 −0	7 −5	9 −2	8 −2	1 −0	6 −3	9 −9	4 −3
7 −3	6 −3	9 −5	5 −0	9 −2	9 −7	9 −0	5 −2	4 −0	7 −3	8 −0	5 −3	6 −0
9 −4	8 −1	5 −2	9 −5	8 −5	8 −1	7 −4	7 −3	9 −9	8 −0	8 −2	7 −7	2 −2
5 −5	8 −3	8 −1	9 −7	8 −0	9 −6	8 −6	4 −0	3 −0	9 −4	9 −8	8 −5	9 −6

52	75	73	65	46	53	51	33	54	98	27	64	65
+45	+17	+65	+68	+47	+89	+77	+68	+50	+18	+56	+97	+88

54	77	51	56	56	27	58	92	34	12	23	85	92
+89	+21	+82	+74	+98	+27	+98	+56	+98	+34	+75	+99	+18

50	92	39	85	79	85	70	91	32	98	75	98	75
+89	+27	+59	+89	+86	+72	+98	+57	+98	+10	+47	+81	+65

25	93	27	89	57	29	84	19	82	47	89	75	72
+93	+85	+72	+98	+57	+35	+79	+83	+75	+89	+83	+27	+48

21	76	26	58	28	50	43	68	93	99	86	76	57
+64	+63	+62	+76	+38	+79	+85	+36	+79	+30	+98	+90	+78

79	44	58	79	45	78	34	74	23	63	28	79	83
+24	+98	+72	+29	+84	+39	+87	+32	+48	+52	+37	+63	+46

42	13	64	23	32	46	34	87	98	59	56	35	60
+97	+93	+86	+97	+69	+89	+86	+78	+96	+38	+76	+72	+51

54	87	85	98	90	97	19	87	93	79	82	78	71
+87	+68	+79	+68	+26	+46	+47	+69	+85	+29	+45	+81	+36

46	75	65	73	28	56	59	51	49	75	68	55	49
+42	+65	+72	+74	+65	+41	+56	+25	+98	+56	+32	+85	+68

97	58	97	59	87	62	65	88	96	57	64	23	22
+95	+21	+89	+25	+23	+28	+56	+24	+75	+64	+28	+94	+25

92	35	30	42	31	43	26	89	90	57	99	75	77
+80	+97	+50	+97	+52	+65	+90	+65	+28	+59	+81	+27	+50

99	57	86	97	69	89	86	87	98	59	76	72	60
−97	−43	−64	−23	−32	−46	−34	−78	−66	−38	−56	−35	−51

87	87	85	98	90	97	47	87	93	79	82	81	71
−54	−68	−79	−68	−26	−46	−19	−69	−85	−29	−45	−78	−36

46	75	72	74	65	56	59	51	98	75	68	85	68
−42	−65	−65	−24	−28	−41	−36	−25	−49	−56	−32	−55	−49

97	58	97	59	87	62	65	88	96	57	64	94	25
−95	−21	−89	−25	−23	−28	−56	−24	−75	−64	−28	−23	−22

92	97	50	97	52	65	90	89	90	59	99	75	77
−80	−35	−30	−42	−31	−43	−26	−65	−28	−57	−81	−27	−50

52	75	73	68	47	89	77	68	54	98	56	97	88
−45	−17	−65	−15	−34	−53	−51	−33	−50	−18	−27	−64	−65

89	77	82	74	98	27	98	92	48	34	75	99	92
−54	−21	−51	−56	−56	−27	−58	−56	−14	−12	−23	−85	−18

89	92	59	89	86	85	98	91	98	98	75	98	75
−50	−27	−39	−59	−79	−72	−70	−57	−32	−10	−47	−81	−65

93	93	72	98	57	35	84	83	82	89	89	75	72
−25	−85	−27	−89	−57	−29	−79	−19	−75	−47	−83	−27	−48

64	76	62	76	38	79	82	68	93	99	98	90	78
−21	−63	−26	−58	−28	−50	−43	−36	−79	−30	−86	−76	−57

79	98	72	79	84	78	87	74	48	63	37	79	83
−24	−44	−58	−29	−49	−39	−34	−32	−23	−52	−28	−63	−46

571 +801	980 +658	579 +701	819 +209	824 +812	761 +740	875 +917	698 +515	570 +687
164 +890	875 +986	834 +596	984 +298	985 +549	872 +889	348 +723	723 +872	175 +186
585 +183	109 +409	920 +850	809 +986	572 +904	390 +670	823 +987	498 +290	109 +809
321 +895	321 +798	654 +585	657 +878	987 +478	513 +363	214 +265	894 +238	891 +665
878 +639	782 +887	749 +268	729 +716	710 +898	984 +417	709 +297	237 +987	562 +597
728 +649	917 +812	981 +981	232 +198	987 +123	394 +987	823 +259	697 +856	298 +398
798 +276	346 +578	982 +347	309 +736	847 +209	239 +391	823 +875	475 +187	348 +676
519 +587	198 +459	239 +869	809 +158	189 +295	938 +687	454 +986	368 +983	723 +287
368 +653	756 +456	875 +215	387 +214	598 +512	759 +255	837 +536	598 +478	678 +785
807 +598	758 +238	583 +775	287 +928	289 +387	398 +592	598 +837	453 +598	279 +275
872 +759	986 +832	798 +759	276 +329	982 +587	679 +298	823 +572	759 +398	823 +769

Copyright © 2003 LinguiSystems, Inc.

824 −812	761 −740	917 −875	698 −515	687 −580	918 −128	549 −274	162 −118	487 −264
985 −549	889 −872	723 −348	872 −661	186 −175	243 −231	983 −673	498 −249	873 −340
904 −572	670 −390	987 −823	498 −290	809 −106	819 −809	971 −875	442 −346	809 −598
987 −478	513 −363	363 −265	894 −238	891 −665	798 −789	721 −697	864 −584	993 −874
842 −898	984 −417	709 −297	237 −112	862 −597	698 −529	536 −198	987 −287	397 −268
987 −123	694 −487	823 −259	997 −656	998 −282	572 −398	938 −237	387 −129	814 −644
847 −209	339 −291	923 −175	475 −187	548 −376	724 −325	887 −390	853 −235	763 −609
289 −195	938 −687	854 −486	768 −383	623 −287	762 −587	657 −312	824 −641	936 −687
598 −512	759 −255	837 −536	598 −478	778 −685	938 −746	764 −355	623 −263	674 −645
389 −287	598 −392	898 −537	553 −498	279 −275	983 −282	754 −375	879 −382	823 −759
982 −587	679 −298	823 −572	759 −398	823 −769	859 −126	823 −798	579 −489	820 −658

words	lamp	the	today
attic	for	when	the
memory	clock	magazine	our
live	write	build	cast
on	doll	first	sink
where	for	travel	celebrate
for	cookie	for	this
today	in	of	clock
orders	this	had	face
quality	the	for	including
since	for	idea	for
for	collectible	was	different
hours	does	the	for
the	the	for	roar
value	the	legend	sound
day	for	by	frame
service	some	for	the
guide	show	the	light
the	from	move	for
cover	for	to	color
items	photos	design	with
love	three	the	create
telephone	back	so	for

throw	future	just	along
that	the	for	the
for	set	want	healthy
to	little	office	diet
room	from	on	could
machine	lamp	for	really
yours	the	when	for
truly	light	find	he
antique	for	for	right
style	sound	that	now
camp	and	stick	where
the	wheels	with	should
for	spring	after	the
statement	touch	few	for
buttons	wood	the	feel
the	base	ago	good
soft	glass	had	can
this	for	for	give
learn	complete	lower	any
why	accent	my	information
breath	use	doctor	when
grow	weather	about	prune
most	the	said	for

large	pinch	the	love
easy	the	statue	right
fact	tips	stone	edge
lot	runners	moss	because
month	them	for	child
excellent	for	winter	for
shorten	our	journal	the
the	the	my	favorite
for	front	the	parents
side	has	friend	the
growing	privacy	porch	for
main	yard	for	return
for	over	out	coming
cane	take	the	gathering
six	not	driving	up
the	will	through	that
each	the	for	for
remove	that	the	watch
tangled	kind	for	black
the	of	once	purple
growth	line	the	season
summer	along	told	looking
for	thinking	the	for

1	2	6	4	4	3	4	1	6	7	9	8	4
9	7	5	2	6	2	6	7	5	7	2	9	7
5	7	5	9	1	8	5	0	8	5	6	2	7
6	9	8	2	7	6	9	4	6	8	0	9	6
2	0	2	7	9	8	7	1	6	8	8	7	1
9	8	5	0	9	6	0	9	2	8	6	7	5
9	8	3	1	5	9	8	1	7	9	0	1	7
4	9	8	1	2	7	9	8	9	5	8	0	9
3	2	8	6	0	9	8	6	8	9	2	7	5
9	8	1	7	2	4	7	1	9	8	4	0	1
9	2	5	0	9	3	8	6	0	9	2	8	2
5	9	8	7	2	9	8	5	9	8	2	5	7
9	8	2	5	6	0	9	3	6	0	4	9	0
5	9	0	5	4	0	7	5	0	9	6	8	3
9	0	8	9	8	1	7	9	8	1	4	9	1
7	4	9	8	1	0	5	9	2	0	6	9	4
3	6	9	5	9	7	0	5	9	7	0	5	0
9	3	5	0	2	9	9	2	0	3	8	3	9
0	8	5	9	0	8	2	7	9	8	2	7	8
9	1	2	4	8	1	7	4	9	0	8	7	2
9	8	7	9	8	6	8	4	0	9	3	8	6
0	3	8	7	0	9	6	0	3	4	9	5	9
3	7	4	9	8	5	7	2	8	5	4	2	5

52	75	73	65	46	53	51	33	54	98	27	64	65
45	17	65	68	47	89	77	68	50	18	56	97	88
54	77	51	56	56	27	58	92	34	12	23	85	92
89	21	82	74	98	27	98	56	98	34	75	99	18
50	92	39	85	79	85	70	91	32	98	75	98	75
89	27	59	89	86	72	98	57	98	10	47	81	65
25	93	27	89	57	29	84	19	82	47	89	75	72
93	85	72	98	57	35	79	83	75	89	83	27	48
21	76	26	58	28	50	43	68	93	99	86	76	57
64	63	62	76	38	79	85	36	79	30	98	90	78
79	44	58	79	45	78	34	74	23	63	28	79	83
24	98	72	29	84	39	87	32	48	52	37	63	46
42	13	64	23	32	46	34	87	98	59	56	35	60
97	93	86	97	69	89	86	78	96	38	76	72	51
54	87	85	98	90	97	19	87	93	79	82	78	71
87	68	79	68	26	46	47	69	85	29	45	81	36
46	75	65	73	28	56	59	51	49	75	68	55	49
42	65	72	74	65	41	56	25	98	56	32	85	68
97	58	97	59	87	62	65	88	96	57	64	23	22
95	21	89	25	23	28	56	24	75	64	28	94	25
92	35	30	42	31	43	26	89	90	57	99	75	57
80	97	50	97	52	65	90	65	28	59	81	27	50
98	27	19	80	74	98	17	50	16	57	86	10	98

571	980	579	819	824	761	875	698	570	918	549	118	264
801	658	701	209	812	740	917	515	687	128	274	162	487
164	875	834	984	985	872	348	723	175	231	673	249	873
890	986	596	298	549	889	723	872	186	243	983	498	340
585	109	920	809	572	390	823	498	109	819	871	209	809
183	409	850	986	904	670	987	290	809	809	875	346	598
321	321	654	657	987	513	214	894	891	789	156	167	819
895	798	585	878	478	363	265	238	665	798	697	584	874
878	782	749	729	710	984	709	237	562	465	236	987	397
639	887	268	716	898	417	297	987	597	529	898	287	268
728	917	981	232	987	394	823	697	298	572	938	187	614
649	812	981	198	123	987	259	856	982	398	237	329	844
798	346	982	309	847	239	823	475	348	724	387	253	763
276	578	347	736	209	391	875	187	676	325	890	835	609
519	198	239	809	189	938	454	368	723	762	357	624	736
587	459	869	158	295	687	986	983	287	587	612	641	687
368	756	875	387	598	759	837	598	678	938	764	623	645
653	456	215	214	512	255	536	478	785	746	355	263	674
807	758	583	287	289	398	598	453	279	983	754	379	823
598	238	775	928	387	592	837	598	275	982	375	982	759
872	986	798	276	982	679	823	759	823	759	823	579	820
759	832	759	329	587	298	572	398	769	826	798	489	658
798	798	376	982	759	828	176	287	965	937	690	878	794

8709	6893	8769	8275	1864	3758	9772	3986	7907	6893	7983	5782	4872
6415	7681	7945	8973	7417	4590	8213	3175	3247	9827	5810	4712	1893
4798	2497	4981	3379	8123	7509	8432	5798	3769	7859	8210	9816	6632
7892	3526	5367	2357	2376	1521	8964	8728	9127	6293	5793	7097	1965
7809	4578	4096	5983	2324	6832	6832	4683	2498	7345	9865	8873	6428
7438	7257	8912	9781	3268	9213	6835	6786	5379	8798	7609	2697	8329
8732	9782	3198	3142	6327	9843	9873	5985	7235	9872	4835	7290	3579
8023	7590	8327	5902	3750	9819	2189	1628	4618	2648	2713	6405	7097
3693	8693	8609	7468	9269	8561	8712	6487	1264	5057	9230	6579	3679
8237	5980	4718	7648	9768	4761	8757	2935	7981	7498	2374	1748	7237
2387	4321	8698	7352	4069	2498	6239	8050	9385	7982	6187	6879	8987
5206	5982	9804	7810	9980	1741	2987	4321	9872	3176	2317	6213	1614
2738	7589	9086	5890	6598	7528	1912	7621	4732	2984	5876	9869	8769
8568	9798	6836	7236	4827	4367	8236	1563	5162	5312	7645	3723	6487
3589	8679	5870	9587	9476	1857	8365	7832	1157	6517	6156	5387	7689
4686	5097	8065	7980	8604	9093	9834	7598	3759	8379	6274	9826	4981
7481	1981	2201	6129	3805	8792	3578	9876	8923	7489	1200	1984	7238
7243	2398	3279	8432	7234	1223	4869	8739	8434	9052	9097	5298	3759
7895	7598	2562	8745	1256	7324	5724	8727	2670	9367	9275	3827	9275
9801	8764	8712	6872	1364	7905	1205	7989	8570	7217	3086	4829	1364
1027	9875	9990	3798	5439	7250	9750	7902	8574	3298	7239	1857	2908
7259	8035	7902	8371	2787	9811	6891	6498	7298	5896	7896	4509	8627
1982	7239	8406	5287	3658	7659	8047	6093	4798	1261	8687	7627	9798

Lucille	Kathleen	Steve	Mary	Frances
Michael	Mary	Genevieve	Michael	Tom
Alexander	Rita	Frank	Peter	Robert
Lillian	Samuel	William	Irene	Augustine
Jane	Betty	Fred	Veronica	Henry
Esther	Bea	Harry	Ethel	Norman
Mary	Michael	John	Michael	Stanley
Dennis	Tom	Mary	Adam	Michael
John	Robert	Margot	Richard	Mary
Henry	Henry	Henry	Gale	Virginia
Kyle	Joseph	Gerald	Ralph	Mary
Robert	Mildred	Michael	Kenneth	Caroline
Ray	John	Frank	Harriet	Maxwell
Howard	Edward	Wallace	Mary	Angelina
Michael	Joyce	Joseph	Michael	Daniel
Caroline	Bernie	Florence	Ethel	Ann
Frederick	John	Daniel	Harry	Marty
Helen	Bessie	Patrick	Dwight	Edward
Mary	Michael	Gregory	Grover	Helen
Bernadine	Helena	Mary	Rudolf	Michael
Mary	Susan	Joe	Ben	Thomas
Joseph	James	Pauline	Alex	Mary
Edwin	William	Michael	Esther	Grace
Thomas	Elizabeth	Veronica	Joseph	Helen
Max	Helen	Evelyn	Marie	Brad
Michael	Ed	Minnie	Louise	Julia
Byron	Ron	Thomas	Walter	Ruth
Charles	Mary	Norma	Michael	Peter
Hugh	Eileen	William	Mary	Anthony
James	Michael	Philip	Marshall	Roy
Helen	Walter	Samuel	Kevin	Harry
Edward	Michael	Joseph	Lillian	Vernon

Michael	Jerome	Helen	Natalie	Sharon
Richard	Dorothy	Arthur	Ellen	Mike
Jeanette	Betty	Donald	Chris	David
Mary	Mildred	Mary	Brian	Michael
Stella	Florence	Angeline	Ricky	Donna
Pauline	Michael	Sam	Sabrina	Donna
Bernice	Franklin	Edward	Kelly	Mary
Gerald	Elijah	Michael	Alan	Kathy
Harry	Michael	Harold	Carrie	Pam
Ruth	Mary	Mary	Stephanie	Claire
Frances	Anna	Gertrude	Mary	Mary
Robert	Charlene	Anthony	Michael	Monica
Michael	Ross	Patricia	Rob	Steve
Ellen	Marie	Kate	Patty	Sally
Kenneth	Charles	Stanley	Connie	Michael
Harriet	Jack	Mary	Janis	Louise
Mary	Michael	Cy	Katie	Karen
Ronald	Lucille	Harry	Dick	Kendra
Margaret	Seymour	Norbert	Ann	Jenny
Jean	Mary	Michael	Connor	Mary
Alfred	Michael	Shirley	Sally	Laura
Robert	Drew	Ruth	Todd	Michelle
Philip	Mary	Julia	Susan	Jeanne
Gerald	Marcella	Stella	Lauren	Laurie
Michael	John	Joyce	Michael	Megan
William	Patrick	George	Charlotte	Tina
John	Eleanor	Adeline	Mary	Michael
Maurice	Michael	Laverne	Christie	Diane
Anna	Ted	Sophie	Tom	Ryan
Mary	Douglas	Mary	Michael	Scott
June	Ronald	Michael	Jack	Wilma
Rose	Dick	Samuel	Catherine	Marion

Mary	Brad	Alex	Jeanne	Christopher
Peter	Tom	Gina	Michael	Rachel
Sean	Jack	Michelle	Venessa	Erin
Sarah	Michael	Olivia	Nell	Marley
Jill	Stephanie	Laura	Megan	Tina
Joe	Kendra	Mary	Jackie	Randy
Mark	Mary	Mark	Bryan	Mary
Hillary	Katherine	Larry	Caitlin	Michael
Michael	Jack	Thomas	Lucy	Nicole
Ellen	Samantha	Michael	Kevin	Melanie
Cheryl	Mary	Matt	Joseph	Patrick
Lisa	Steven	Madeline	Mary	Megan
Christy	Jeremy	Caroline	Spencer	Tim
Tom	Kyle	Mac	Joe	Christie
Phil	Michael	Tony	Michael	Margaret
Kevin	Kendra	Chloe	Eddie	Lauren
Mary	Thomas	Katie	Allie	Eddie
Grace	Julie	Malcolm	Madeline	Christine
Roberto	Frank	Mary	Charlie	Michael
Peter	Grant	Joanne	Amanda	Mary
Tim	Brian	Danielle	Lara	Scott
Patrick	Michael	Michael	Jasmine	Darla
Michael	Ryan	Colleen	Molly	Bobby
Matthew	Mary	Nikki	Nick	Teddy
Billy	Max	Alexa	Mary	Luke
Allison	Daniel	Joey	Sarah	Cathy
Quinn	Karen	Andrew	Michael	Jocelyn
Jonathan	Colleen	Will	Julie	Pete
Emily	Michael	Rebecca	Melanie	Elena
Mary	Jeffrey	Monica	Neal	Lisa
Maggie	Rachel	Adam	Richard	Larry
Connor	Connor	Mary	Kathy	Maria

Michael	Stacey	Anita	Tom	Irene
Dorothy	Janis	Sam	Bud	Helene
Mary	Sandy	Lois	Mary	Agnes
Karen	Dennis	Fred	Joan	Shirley
Jill	Betsy	Emily	Angela	Maureen
Louis	Michael	Judy	Shannon	Corrine
George	Helen	Mary	Michael	Helen
Eileen	Dick	Nancy	Jerome	Diana
Patricia	Martha	Russ	Marguerite	Mary
Barbara	Marvin	Felix	Audrey	John
Oscar	Lucille	Melissa	Rebecca	Michael
Daniel	Mary	Marlene	Melvin	Leonard
Michael	Cesar	Michael	Carlos	James
Juliet	Noah	Leo	Laurie	Vince
Gina	Harold	Vicki	Mary	Scott
David	Loraine	Clifford	Harold	Dean
Mary	Michael	Dennis	Douglas	Hector
Sylvia	Carlos	Alice	Michael	Gertrude
Josie	Michael	Rose	Judith	Ernesto
Rosemarie	Alvin	Ellen	Karen	Jennifer
Al	Heather	Mary	Rosie	Tyrone
Joe	Charles	Florence	Caroline	Mary
Joyce	Theresa	Sharon	Allison	Michael
Denise	Mary	Julie	Norm	Delores
Paul	Phyllis	Stanley	Samuel	Everett
Michael	Mario	Michael	Martha	Vivian
Bernadette	Cora	Dorothy	Teresa	Beth
Stephen	Gladys	Barry	Mary	Sandra
John	Cindy	Amy	Peggy	Rita
Mary	Albert	Tim	Michael	Victoria
Jan	Michael	Ken	Joy	Hilary
Debbie	Joan	Lyle	Donna	Annette

Distractions Worksheet

Name: _____ Date: _____

Task	Distractions Present	Modifications

BIG	LITTLE	big	little	LITTLE	big	BIG
LITTLE	big	LITTLE	big	little	little	big
BIG	LITTLE	big	BIG	LITTLE	big	little
little	LITTLE	big	BIG	LITTLE	big	LITTLE
big	little	BIG	LITTLE	big	LITTLE	big
little	little	big	BIG	LITTLE	big	BIG
LITTLE	big	little	little	LITTLE	LITTLE	big
BIG	LITTLE	big	LITTLE	big	little	BIG
LITTLE	big	LITTLE	big	little	little	big
BIG	LITTLE	big	BIG	little	BIG	LITTLE
big	LITTLE	big	little	little	big	BIG
LITTLE	big	LITTLE	big	little	BIG	LITTLE
big	LITTLE	big	little	little	big	BIG
LITTLE	big	BIG	little	BIG	LITTLE	big
LITTLE	big	little	LITTLE	big	BIG	LITTLE
big	LITTLE	big	little	little	big	BIG
LITTLE	big	BIG	LITTLE	big	little	little
big	BIG	little	BIG	LITTLE	big	LITTLE
big	little	LITTLE	BIG	BIG	LITTLE	big
LITTLE	big	little	little	big	BIG	LITTLE
LITTLE	big	little	little	big	BIG	LITTLE
big	BIG	little	BIG	LITTLE	BIG	little
LITTLE	big	LITTLE	big	little	little	big

Fat	Skinny	Fat	**Skinny**	**Fat**
Skinny	Fat	**Skinny**	Fat	Skinny
Fat	**Skinny**	**Fat**	**Skinny**	Fat
Fat	Skinny	Fat	Skinny	**Fat**
Skinny	Fat	**Skinny**	**Fat**	Fat
Skinny	**Fat**	Skinny	Fat	Skinny
Fat	**Skinny**	Skinny	**Fat**	**Skinny**
Fat	Skinny	**Fat**	Skinny	Fat
Skinny	Fat	Skinny	Fat	**Skinny**
Fat	**Skinny**	Skinny	**Fat**	Skinny
Skinny	Skinny	Fat	**Skinny**	Fat
Fat	Fat	Skinny	Fat	Skinny
Fat	Skinny	**Fat**	**Skinny**	Fat
Fat	Fat	Skinny	Fat	Skinny
Skinny	**Fat**	**Skinny**	Fat	Fat
Skinny	**Fat**	Skinny	**Fat**	Skinny
Fat	**Skinny**	Fat	Skinny	Fat
Skinny	Fat	**Skinny**	Fat	**Skinny**
Fat	Skinny	Fat	**Skinny**	Fat
Skinny	**Fat**	Skinny	**Fat**	Fat
Fat	Skinny	**Fat**	**Skinny**	**Skinny**
Skinny	Skinny	**Fat**	Skinny	Fat
Skinny	Fat	Skinny	Fat	**Fat**

Print	Cursive	Print	Cursive	Cursive	Print
Cursive	Print	Cursive	Cursive	Print	Cursive
Cursive	Print	Cursive	Cursive	Cursive	Print
Print	Cursive	Print	Cursive	Cursive	Print
Cursive	Print	Cursive	Cursive	Print	Cursive
Cursive	Print	Cursive	Cursive	Cursive	Print
Print	Cursive	Print	Cursive	Cursive	Print
Cursive	Print	Cursive	Cursive	Print	Cursive
Cursive	Print	Cursive	Print	Cursive	Print
Cursive	Cursive	Print	Cursive	Print	Cursive
Cursive	Print	Cursive	Cursive	Cursive	Cursive
Print	Cursive	Cursive	Print	Cursive	Print
Cursive	Print	Cursive	Cursive	Print	Cursive
Print	Cursive	Cursive	Print	Cursive	Cursive
Cursive	Cursive	Print	Cursive	Cursive	Print
Cursive	Print	Cursive	Cursive	Print	Cursive
Cursive	Print	Cursive	Print	Cursive	Print
Cursive	Cursive	Print	Cursive	Print	Cursive
Cursive	Print	Cursive	Cursive	Print	Cursive
Print	Cursive	Cursive	Print	Cursive	Print
Cursive	Print	Print	Cursive	Cursive	Print
Cursive	Print	Cursive	Cursive	Print	Cursive
Cursive	Print	Cursive	Cursive	Cursive	Print

 Copyright © 2003 LinguiSystems, Inc.

BOLD	LIGHT	BOLD	LIGHT	**LIGHT**	BOLD	**BOLD**
LIGHT	**LIGHT**	BOLD	LIGHT	LIGHT	**LIGHT**	BOLD
LIGHT	BOLD	LIGHT	**LIGHT**	BOLD	**BOLD**	LIGHT
BOLD	**LIGHT**	BOLD	LIGHT	**LIGHT**	BOLD	**BOLD**
LIGHT	BOLD	LIGHT	**LIGHT**	BOLD	**BOLD**	LIGHT
BOLD	**LIGHT**	BOLD	**LIGHT**	BOLD	LIGHT	LIGHT
LIGHT	BOLD	**LIGHT**	BOLD	LIGHT	**LIGHT**	BOLD
BOLD	**LIGHT**	**BOLD**	LIGHT	BOLD	BOLD	LIGHT
LIGHT	BOLD	**BOLD**	LIGHT	BOLD	LIGHT	**LIGHT**
BOLD	**BOLD**	LIGHT	**BOLD**	LIGHT	BOLD	LIGHT
BOLD	LIGHT	LIGHT	**LIGHT**	BOLD	**LIGHT**	**BOLD**
LIGHT	BOLD	BOLD	LIGHT	**LIGHT**	BOLD	**BOLD**
LIGHT	BOLD	LIGHT	**LIGHT**	BOLD	**BOLD**	LIGHT
BOLD	LIGHT	**LIGHT**	BOLD	**BOLD**	LIGHT	**BOLD**
LIGHT	LIGHT	LIGHT	**LIGHT**	BOLD	**LIGHT**	**BOLD**
LIGHT	BOLD	BOLD	LIGHT	**LIGHT**	BOLD	**BOLD**
LIGHT	BOLD	**LIGHT**	BOLD	LIGHT	**LIGHT**	BOLD
BOLD	**LIGHT**	**BOLD**	**LIGHT**	BOLD	**LIGHT**	BOLD
LIGHT	LIGHT	**LIGHT**	BOLD	LIGHT	**BOLD**	LIGHT
BOLD	BOLD	LIGHT	BOLD	**BOLD**	LIGHT	**BOLD**
LIGHT	LIGHT	LIGHT	**LIGHT**	LIGHT	**BOLD**	LIGHT
BOLD	**LIGHT**	BOLD	LIGHT	**LIGHT**	**BOLD**	LIGHT

Task Combination Worksheet

Name:	Date:

Tasks	Appropriate Combinations	Times	Reminders

Copyright © 2003 LinguiSystems, Inc.

52 +45	75 +17	73 +65	65 +68	46 +47	53 +89	51 +77	33 +68	54 +50	98 +18	27 +56	64 +97	65 +88
94 −89	77 −21	81 −42	76 −54	96 −58	27 −27	98 −58	92 −56	94 −38	32 −14	73 −25	95 −89	92 −18
50 +89	92 +27	39 +59	85 +89	79 +86	85 +72	70 +98	91 +57	32 +98	98 +10	75 +47	98 +81	75 +65
95 −23	93 −85	77 −22	99 −88	57 −57	39 −25	84 −79	89 −13	82 −75	87 −49	89 −83	75 −27	72 −48
21 +64	76 +63	26 +62	58 +76	28 +38	50 +79	43 +85	68 +36	93 +79	99 +30	86 +98	76 +90	57 +78
79 −24	94 −48	78 −52	79 −29	85 −44	78 −39	84 −37	74 −32	43 −28	63 −52	68 −37	89 −63	83 −46
42 +97	13 +93	64 +86	23 +97	32 +69	46 +89	34 +86	87 +78	98 +96	59 +38	56 +76	35 +72	60 +51
84 −57	87 −68	85 −29	98 −68	90 −26	97 −46	49 −17	87 −69	93 −35	79 −29	62 −45	88 −71	71 −36
46 +42	75 +65	65 +72	73 +74	28 +65	56 +41	59 +56	51 +25	49 +98	75 +56	68 +32	55 +85	49 +68
97 −95	58 −21	97 −89	59 −25	87 −23	62 −28	65 −56	88 −24	96 −75	67 −34	64 −28	93 −24	51 −25
92 +80	35 +97	30 +50	42 +97	31 +52	43 +65	26 +90	89 +65	90 +28	57 +59	99 +81	75 +27	77 +50

Alternating Attention Math

92 +80	97 −35	50 +30	97 −42	52 +31	65 −43	90 +26	89 −65	90 +28	59 −57	99 +81	75 −27	77 +50
52 −45	75 +17	73 −65	68 +15	47 −34	89 +53	77 −51	68 +33	54 −50	98 +18	56 −27	97 +64	88 −65
89 +54	77 −21	82 −51	74 +56	98 −56	27 +27	98 −58	92 +56	48 −14	34 +12	75 −23	99 +85	92 −18
89 +50	92 −27	59 +39	89 −59	86 +79	85 −72	98 +70	91 −57	98 +32	98 −10	75 +47	98 −81	75 +65
93 −25	93 +85	72 −27	98 +89	57 −57	35 +29	84 −79	83 +19	82 −75	89 +47	89 −83	75 +27	72 −48
64 +21	76 −63	62 +26	76 −58	38 +28	79 −50	82 +43	68 −36	93 +79	99 −30	98 +86	90 −76	78 +57
79 −24	98 +44	72 −58	79 +29	84 −49	78 +39	87 −34	74 +32	48 −23	63 +52	37 −28	79 +63	83 −46
99 +97	57 −43	86 +64	97 −23	69 +32	89 −46	86 +34	87 −78	98 +66	59 −38	76 +56	72 −35	60 +51
87 −54	87 +68	85 −79	98 +68	90 −26	97 +46	47 −19	87 +69	93 −85	79 +29	82 −45	81 +78	71 −36
46 +42	75 −65	72 +65	74 −24	65 +28	56 −41	59 +36	51 −25	98 +49	75 −56	68 +32	85 −55	68 +49
97 −95	58 +21	97 −89	59 +25	87 −23	62 +28	65 −56	88 +24	96 −75	57 +64	64 −28	94 +23	25 −22

Alternating Attention Math

50 +89	72 −27	39 x 9	85 +89	79 +86	85 x 7	70 −61	89 x 6	32 −11	98 +22	75 +27	98 −30	75 −42
63 +65	22 x 7	45 x 2	92 +36	73 −27	61 +55	68 +43	50 −28	27 x 6	31 −28	42 +27	50 +68	22 −18
48 +21	98 −63	33 x 6	57 x 8	52 +28	98 −50	82 +43	68 −26	84 +79	62 −30	98 x 6	90 −76	87 x 7
79 x 4	56 +44	83 −58	25 +29	92 −49	78 x 9	87 x 4	65 +32	32 −23	61 −52	87 +28	79 +63	83 x 6
69 +27	95 −43	86 x 4	85 −23	34 +32	67 x 4	68 x 3	67 −16	98 x 6	68 −38	76 +56	72 x 3	50 +51
87 −54	87 −68	85 −79	98 +68	80 x 6	17 x 3	47 −19	87 +69	93 −85	79 +39	72 −45	81 +68	61 x 6
46 x 4	75 x 5	72 −65	64 +24	55 +28	56 −41	69 x 6	51 x 5	98 −49	75 −56	68 +32	58 x 2	68 x 9
87 −59	48 +21	67 −28	59 x 2	87 x 8	62 +28	65 −36	78 +24	46 −24	50 x 9	64 −28	94 +23	25 −22
54 x 7	68 −32	32 +34	57 +20	93 −54	47 x 7	56 x 6	31 +54	17 −10	27 +27	48 −29	62 x 4	91 x 3
64 +84	27 x 6	31 x 9	12 +82	88 −12	73 x 7	41 x 6	53 +43	67 +19	89 −71	19 +73	42 x 2	77 +63

Simultaneous Tasks Worksheet

Name:	Date:

Simultaneous Tasks	Problems	Modifications

Odds   **Evens**

1	2	6	4	4	3	4	1	6
7	9	8	4	9	7	5	2	6
2	6	7	5	7	2	9	7	5
7	5	9	1	8	5	0	8	5
6	2	7	6	9	8	2	7	6
9	4	6	8	0	9	6	2	0
2	7	9	8	7	1	6	8	8
7	1	9	8	5	0	9	6	0
9	2	8	6	7	5	9	8	3
1	5	9	8	1	7	9	0	1
7	4	9	8	1	2	7	9	8
9	5	8	0	9	3	2	8	6
0	9	8	6	8	9	2	7	5
9	8	1	7	2	4	7	1	9
8	4	0	1	5	9	8	1	7
9	0	1	7	4	9	8	1	2
9	8	9	5	8	0	9	3	8
9	2	7	5	9	8	1	7	2
4	7	1	9	8	4	0	1	5
8	0	9	3	8	2	7	5	9
8	1	7	2	4	7	1	9	8

Odds   Evens

52	75	73	65	46	53	51	33	54
98	27	64	65	45	17	65	68	47
89	77	68	50	18	56	97	88	54
77	51	56	56	27	58	92	34	12
23	85	92	89	21	82	74	98	27
98	56	98	34	75	99	18	50	92
39	85	79	85	70	91	32	98	75
98	75	89	27	59	89	86	72	98
57	98	10	47	81	65	25	93	27
89	57	29	84	19	82	47	89	75
72	93	85	72	98	57	35	79	83
75	89	83	27	48	21	76	26	58
28	50	43	68	93	99	86	76	57
64	63	62	76	38	79	85	36	79
30	98	90	78	79	44	58	79	45
78	34	74	23	63	28	79	83	24
98	72	29	84	39	87	32	48	52
37	63	46	42	13	64	23	32	46
34	87	98	59	56	35	60	97	93
86	97	69	89	86	78	96	38	76
72	51	78	79	44	58	79	45	78

Odds   Evens

980	579	819	824	761	875	698	570	918
549	118	264	801	658	701	209	812	740
917	515	687	128	274	162	487	164	875
834	984	985	872	348	723	175	231	673
249	873	890	986	596	298	549	889	723
872	186	243	983	498	340	585	109	920
809	572	390	823	498	109	819	871	209
809	183	409	850	986	904	670	987	290
809	809	875	346	598	321	321	654	657
987	513	214	894	891	789	156	167	819
895	798	585	878	478	363	265	238	665
798	697	584	874	878	782	749	729	710
984	709	237	562	465	236	987	397	639
887	268	716	898	417	297	987	597	529
898	287	268	728	917	981	232	987	394
823	697	298	572	938	187	614	649	812
981	198	123	987	259	856	982	398	237
329	844	798	346	982	309	847	239	823
475	348	724	387	253	763	276	578	347
736	209	391	875	187	676	325	890	835
609	519	198	239	809	189	938	454	368

accident	bend	cabinet	contact
account	bill	calf	corn
act	bit	can	count
admit	blank	cap	counter
appreciate	block	case	court
arm	blow	cast	cover
ash	blue	center	crab
average	bluff	change	crack
back	board	channel	crane
bail	boil	charge	creep
ball	bolt	charm	cricket
band	bore	check	critical
bangs	boss	chest	crop
bank	bow	china	cross
bar	bowl	chip	curb
bark	box	chop	dampen
base	brake	class	dart
baste	brand	clip	dash
bat	brick	club	date
batter	bridge	clutch	deal
beam	brief	coat	deck
bear	buck	cold	decline
beat	buckle	colon	dip
bed	bug	company	direction
bell	bump	complex	dock
belt	cable	concentration	down

draft	flat	hail	lace
draw	float	ham	land
dress	flounder	hamper	lap
drill	flush	hand	last
drop	fly	hard	lean
duck	foil	harp	leaves
dull	fool	hatch	left
ear	foot	haze	letter
egg	fork	head	lie
elder	foul	hide	light
endorse	frame	hike	like
engage	free	hit	limb
eye	fret	hood	line
face	fudge	host	lip
fair	game	ice	loaf
fall	gear	incline	lock
fan	general	iron	lodge
fast	glasses	jack	log
felt	grade	jam	long
file	grate	jar	lounge
film	graze	jerk	maroon
fine	grease	judge	mask
finish	green	key	mass
fire	grill	kid	match
firm	groom	kind	mate
fit	ground	knock	mean
flag	gum	knot	meet

might	period	press	roast
milk	permit	prime	rock
mine	pet	prop	room
mint	physical	prune	rose
miss	pick	punch	round
mold	pinch	pupil	row
mole	pit	purse	ruler
mug	pitch	quack	run
nail	pitcher	quality	rung
nap	place	quarter	runner
negative	plain	race	safe
novel	plane	racket	sage
nut	plant	range	saw
orange	plate	rare	scale
order	play	rash	school
organ	plot	rate	seal
pack	poach	rattle	season
page	point	rear	second
palm	poker	record	select
panel	pole	reflect	sentence
pants	pool	refrain	set
park	pop	relish	shake
part	port	report	share
pass	position	rest	sharp
patient	positive	rich	shed
pen	post	right	sheet
perch	pound	ring	shock

shop	stalk	tap	watch
short	stall	tape	wave
shot	stamp	temple	well
sight	stand	tense	whip
sign	staple	tick	will
sink	star	tie	yard
slide	state	tip	
slip	stay	tire	
slug	steer	toast	
snap	stick	toll	
soil	still	top	
sole	stock	toy	
solution	strain	track	
sound	strand	trail	
space	straw	train	
spade	strike	truck	
spare	strip	trunk	
speaker	stroke	tumbler	
spell	stump	tune	
spoke	sty	turkey	
spot	submarine	turn	
spring	suspect	type	
square	swallow	uniform	
squash	switch	utter	
stable	tag	vault	
staff	tail	vice	
stage	tank	wake	

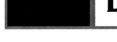

Begin with the letter *A* and draw a line to the number *1*. Continue by drawing a line to *B*, then *2*, and so on, alternating letters and numbers, in order.

A

I

E

6   5   J

B

F

1

7

8

D

3   10

4   G

C

9

H   2

Begin with the letter *A* and draw a line to the number *1*. Continue by drawing a line to *B*, then *2*, and so on, alternating letters and numbers, in order.

4

A

F

H

J

D

1

8

9

2

G

I

E

10

5

7

C

6

B

3

Begin with the number 1 and connect all the odd numbers in order. Then connect the highest odd number to the lowest even number and connect all the even numbers in order.

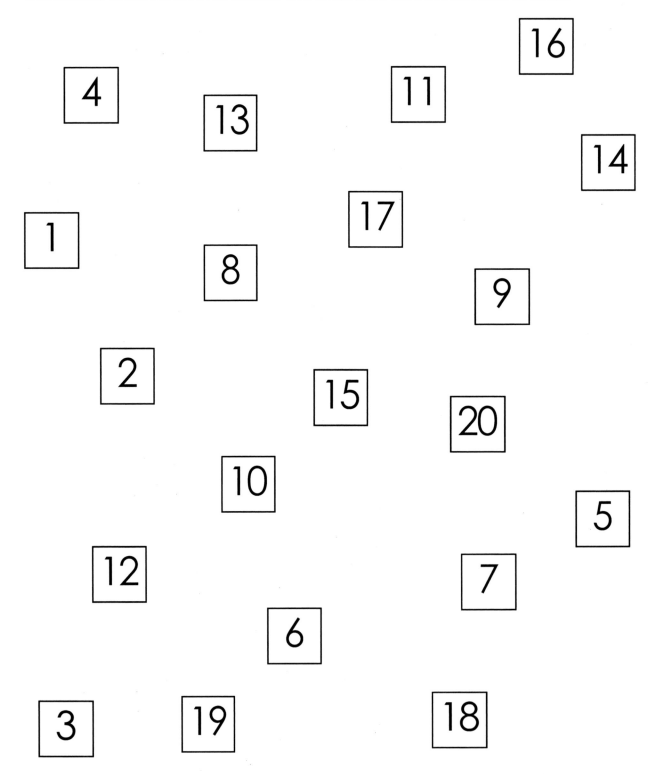

Begin with the number 1 in the square and connect it to the number 1 in the circle. Connect the number 1 in the circle to the number 2 in the square and continue connecting numbers in order, alternating between the same number in the two different shapes.

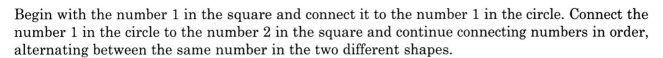

Only red cards

Only black cards

Only even cards

Only odd cards

Only face cards

Only female face cards

Only male face cards

Only spades

Only clubs

Only hearts

Only diamonds

Only even red cards

Only odd red cards

Only even black cards

Only odd black cards

Only even spades

Only odd spades

Only even clubs

Only odd clubs

Only even hearts

Only odd hearts

Only even diamonds

Only odd diamonds

Only even red and odd black cards

Only odd red and even black cards

Only spades and hearts

Only spades and diamonds

Only clubs and hearts

Only clubs and diamonds

Only even cards and face cards

Only odd cards and face cards

Only red cards and Queens

Only black cards and Queens

Only even cards and Kings

Only odd cards and Kings

Only Aces and 2s

Plan–Execute–Repair

The essence of executive functions may be expressed in three words: *Plan–Execute–Repair*. These words will become a mantra for patients. Patients will learn to ask themselves the following questions as they move through the Plan-Execute-Repair phases:

➤ **Plan:** What am I trying to accomplish?

➤ **Plan:** What are the necessary steps?

➤ **Plan:** What is the sequence of these steps?

➤ **Plan:** How long will each step take?

➤ **Plan/Execute:** How and when do I start?

➤ **Execute:** How will I persevere with the task?

➤ **Execute/Repair:** What could possibly go wrong?

➤ **Repair:** How is my plan moving along? Do I need to alter the plan?

➤ **Execute:** How will I know when I'm finished?

➤ **Repair:** What would I do differently next time?

➤ **Repair:** What would I do the same next time?

Helpful Hint: Business publications often contain articles and forms on project management that can be kept as examples and shared with patients.

A personal organizational system will play an important role in the Plan-Execute-Repair phase. Each target task will be housed in the system where it is easily located for frequent use. Some organizational systems come with their own project management sections and forms but others do not. Provide the patient with the **Planning Form** on page 166 if needed. An example is shown on the next page.

"Plan" Phase:
What am I trying to accomplish?

➤ Begin with a well-defined task that has an explicit end result and straightforward steps toward this result. Employ the patient's schedule and to-do lists to determine an appropriate task. Consider Phase 7 (Prioritizing) of Time Management in selecting a task.

➤ Have the patient clearly state the goal and write it in the "Task" box. For example, what appears in the organizational system as "Bob's Birthday" should be refined to "Have Bob's birthday gift ready by Saturday evening." Ask the patient to write the specific task, which is the end result, in the organizational system.

Planning Form			
Task: Have Bob's birthday gift ready by Saturday evening.			
Steps	**Completion Schedule**	**✔**	**Feedback**

"Plan" Phase:
What are the necessary steps?

➤ Have the client work backwards from the desired end result and pick out each individual step involved in reaching the goal. Focus on writing as many options and ideas as possible. Here are some sample steps to consider:
• Wrap gift.
• Buy gift.
• Go to the store.
• Schedule time to go to the store.
• Brainstorm gift ideas.
• Decide on a budget.

➤ Each of the steps listed above has ancillary components that need to be listed:
1. Wrap gift.
    ✔ Have wrap, ribbon, box, and tape on hand.
    ✔ Shop if these supplies are unavailable.
    ✔ Schedule time to shop.
2. Buy gift.

156

Copyright © 2003 LinguiSystems, Inc.

3. Go to the store.
    ✔ Drive, park, shop, check out, and drive home.
    ✔ Have money — go to the bank.
        • Schedule time to go to the bank.
4. Brainstorm gift ideas.
    ✔ Look online — check delivery times and fees.
    ✔ Look in catalogs — check delivery times and fees.
    ✔ Look around at the mall.
        • Schedule time to go to the mall.
    ✔ Talk to friends about ideas.
        • Schedule time to talk to friends.
5. Decide on a budget.
    ✔ Balance checkbook.

What appeared on paper to be a single activity, "Bob's birthday," is actually a 15-20 step process. Patients with executive function disorders fail to recognize all the components of the task and, therefore, fail to schedule adequate time to complete each of the steps.

The most appropriate treatment tasks for identifying specific steps of a larger task are found within the patient's real-life activities. Once meaningful activities have been identified, manipulate the difficulty of this phase by doing the following:

➤ **Identifying Critical Steps:** Provide the patient with a variety of steps, both critical and unrelated to the target task and ask the patient to identify which steps are components of the target task and which are not. For example, provide the patient with these steps and ask him or her to identify which ones are related to "having Bob's birthday gift ready by Saturday evening":

   • deciding on a budget
   • getting gasoline for the car
   • shopping for the gift
   • wrapping the gift
   • baking a cake
   • looking for decorations

➤ **Critical Step Omission:** Provide the patient with a variety of steps related to the target task, omit several key components, and ask the patient to identify the missing steps. On the following page is an incomplete list of steps for buying and wrapping a birthday gift. Have your patient fill in the missing steps.

1. Wrap gift.
   ✔ Have wrap, ribbon, box, and tape on hand.
   ✔ _____
   ✔ _____
2. Buy gift.
3. Go to the store.
   ✔ _____
   ✔ Have money — go to the bank.
      · Schedule time to go to the bank.
4. Brainstorm gift ideas.
   ✔ Look online — check delivery times and fees.
   ✔ _____
   ✔ Look around at the mall.
      · Schedule time to go to the mall.
   ✔ _____
      · Schedule time to talk to friends.
5. Decide on a budget.
   ✔ _____

➤ **Critical Step Generation:** Provide the patient with the target task and the number of steps and sub-steps involved in outline form. Then have the patient fill in the steps.

Task: Buying a birthday gift

1. _____
   ✔ _____
   ✔ _____
   ✔ _____
2. _____
3. _____
   ✔ _____
   ✔ _____
      · _____
4. _____
   ✔ _____
   ✔ _____
   ✔ _____
      · _____

 ✔ _____
 • _____

5. _____
 ✔ _____

Occasionally patients will require more clinical practice to master the ability to generate all the steps of a task. Specific practice examples are provided on the **Task Steps Activities** on pages 167-170.

▣ **Planning Form**

Task:	Have Bob's birthday gift ready by Saturday evening.

Steps	Completion Schedule	✔	Feedback
Balance checkbook.			
Decide budget.			
Schedule time to go to the mall.			
Schedule time to talk to friends.			
Look in catalogs—check delivery times and fees.			
Look online—check delivery times and fees.			
Look around at the mall.			
Talk to friends about ideas.			
Schedule time to go to the bank.			
Go to the bank.			
Drive to the store and park.			
Shop and check out—ask for a box.			
Buy wrap and ribbon.			
Drive home.			
Wrap gift.			

"Plan" Phase:
What is the sequence of these steps?

The next task is to decide on the order of the steps needed to accomplish the goal. Have the patient consider which steps need to be completed prior to others. Encourage the patient to combine steps when appropriate, such as shop for gift wrap during the same time as shopping for the gift.

Again, the most appropriate treatment tasks for specific step sequences are found within the patient's real-life activities. The level of difficulty for sequencing can be manipulated by doing the following:

➤ **Critical Step Omission:** Provide the patient with a variety of steps related to the target task, omit several key components, and ask the patient to identify the missing steps.

➤ **Critical Step Generation:** Provide the patient with the target task and the number of steps and sub-steps involved in outline form. Then have the patient fill in the steps.

There are many available activities to address sequencing in isolation:
➤ letters into words
➤ words into sentences
➤ sentences into paragraphs
➤ number patterns

Occasionally patients will require more clinical practice to master sequencing of steps in functional activities. Examples are provided in the **Task Sequencing Activities** on page 171.

The end product, steps, and the sequence of the steps should be clearly written in the patient's organizational system and carried with the patient. This provides a "blueprint" of the plan.

"Plan" Phase:
How long will each step take?

Utilize the **Time Estimation Worksheet** on page 72 if the patient has not yet mastered this skill. Have the patient analyze the time requirements for every step and calculate the total time needed to complete the task, as in the example on the right.

"Plan" and "Execute" Phases:
How and when do I start?

Once the length of time each step will take has been established, begin to work with the patient in determining where that time is available in the schedule. For example, if shopping will take 2 hours, but the patient doesn't have 2 hours free the several days prior to the due date, this dilemma needs to be known prior to the day before the due date. Once times are slotted, the patient will then write component steps into his or her daily and weekly schedule and on daily and weekly to-do lists. The example on the next page includes these considerations.

Planning Form

Task:	Have Bob's birthday gift ready by Saturday evening.

Steps	Completion Schedule	✔	Feedback
Balance checkbook.	15 minutes		
Decide budget.	3 minutes		
Schedule time to go to the mall.	5 minutes		
Schedule time to talk to friends.	with above		
Look in catalogs—check delivery times and fees.	15 minutes		
Look online—check delivery times and fees.	30 minutes		
Look around at the mall.	20 minutes		
Talk to friends about ideas.	20 minutes		
Schedule time to go to the bank.	with third item		
Go to the bank.	20 minutes		
Drive to the store and park.	10 minutes		
Shop and check out—ask for a box.	30 minutes		
Buy wrap and ribbon.	with above		
Drive home.	10 minutes		
Wrap gift.	10 minutes		

Planning Form

Task: Have Bob's birthday gift ready by Saturday evening.

Steps	Completion Schedule	✔	Feedback
Balance checkbook.	15 minutes Sunday afternoon		
Decide budget.	3 minutes Sunday afternoon		
Schedule time to go to the mall.	5 minutes Monday morning		
Schedule time to talk to friends.	with above		
Look in catalogs—check delivery times and fees.	15 minutes Monday evening		
Look online—check delivery times and fees.	30 minutes Monday evening		
Look around at the mall.	No time—omit		
Talk to friends about ideas.	20 minutes Wed. afternoon		
Schedule time to go to the bank.	with third item Monday morning		
Go to the bank.	20 minutes Leave Fri. 5:00pm		
Drive to the store and park.	10 minutes Friday		
Shop and check out—ask for a box.	30 minutes Friday		
Buy wrap and ribbon.	with above Friday		
Drive home.	10 minutes Fri. 8:00pm		
Wrap gift.	10 minutes Sat. 3:00 pm		

Determining the exact date and time to begin, combined with dividing the target task into smaller, manageable components, can help break the inertia frequently described by patients with executive function disorders. Instruct the patient to check off each step when it is accomplished.

The **Time Estimation Worksheet** on page 72 is useful initially. Have the patient use a clock or watch alarm as a reminder of when to start or stop an activity.

Utilizing the patient's target tasks and schedules is the most effective form of practice. Occasionally, patients will require more structured practice. **Task Sequencing Activities** can be found on page 171 and **Task Combination Activities** are on page 172.

"Execute" Phase: How will I persevere with the task?

What are the requirements of attention for each step of the process? Ask the patient to analyze each step for possible challenges to each level of attention.

➤ Does any step require the patient to pay attention for a longer period of time than he or she is capable of? If so, the patient will need to break the step into multiple phases.

➤ Does any step tax the patient's selective attention? Are there distractions that can be minimized or eliminated prior to initiating the step?

➤ Does any step require the patient to divide or alternate attention beyond personal limits?

The example on the next page displays some of the challenges mentioned above and presents ways to address them.

Planning Form

Task: Have Bob's birthday gift ready by Saturday evening.

Steps	Completion Schedule	✔	Feedback
Balance checkbook. **Need Silence**	15 minutes Sunday afternoon		
Decide budget.	3 minutes Sunday afternoon		
Schedule time to go to the mall.	5 minutes Monday morning		
Schedule time to talk to friends.	with above		
Look in catalogs—check delivery times and fees.	15 minutes Monday evening		
Look online—check delivery times and fees. **Set alarm to limit to 30 minutes.**	30 minutes Monday evening		
Talk to friends about ideas.	20 minutes Wed. afternoon		
Schedule time to go to the bank.	with third item Monday morning		
Go to the bank.	20 minutes Leave Fri. 5:00pm		
Drive to the store and park.	10 minutes Friday		
Shop and check out—ask for a box. Buy wrap and ribbon. **Keep list handy to stay on track.**	30 minutes Friday		
Drive home.	10 minutes Fri. 8:00pm		
Wrap gift.	10 minutes Sat. 3:00 pm		

"Execute" and "Repair" Phases: What could possibly go wrong?

A complete list of pitfalls for any task could be immense! Instead, have your patient stick with the most likely interferences and anticipate ways to work through them. Here are some examples:

➤ The wanted gift was not available for 2 weeks:
  • Decide this is the perfect gift and give Bob an "IOU" due in two weeks.
  • Find a different gift.

➤ The item doesn't fit in the box available:
  • Buy many different-sized boxes at once.
  • Use a gift bag instead.

➤ Your car is scheduled for repairs the week you plan to shop for Bob's gift:
  · Change shopping schedule.
  · Change car repair appointment.
  · Borrow or rent a car for the day.
  · Take public transportation.
      ✔ Does it go where you need to go? Can you shop elsewhere?

Have the patient modify the schedule to allow for the likely interruptions and schedule backup plans.

Planning Form

Task: Have Bob's birthday gift ready by Saturday evening.

Steps	Completion Schedule	✔	Feedback
Balance checkbook. *Need Silence*	15 minutes Sunday afternoon		
Decide budget.	3 minutes Sunday afternoon		
Schedule time to go to the mall.	5 minutes Monday morning		
Schedule time to talk to friends.	with above		
Look in catalogs—check delivery times and fees.	15 minutes Monday evening		Bob said he has trouble with returns not in town—don't use catalogs.
Look online—check delivery times and fees. *Set alarm to limit to 30 minutes.*	30 minutes Monday evening		Got off task looking at other items not related to gift—consider less than 30 minutes and use a louder alarm.
Talk to friends about ideas.	20 minutes Wed. afternoon		
Schedule time to go to the bank.	with third item Monday morning		
Go to the bank.	20 minutes Leave Fri. 5:00pm		
Drive to the store and park.	10 minutes Friday		
Shop and check out—ask for a box. Buy wrap and ribbon. *Keep list handy to stay on track.*	30 minutes Friday		
Drive home.	10 minutes Fri. 8:00pm		
Wrap gift.	10 minutes Sat. 3:00 pm		

"Repair" Phase: How is my plan moving along? Do I need to alter the plan?

Continuous analysis of the plan, its steps, and the sequence is mandatory. The patient needs to be in the repair phase throughout, asking questions such as these:

➤ Is the end product still the same?

➤ Are there additional steps?

➤ Can some steps be eliminated?

➤ Is the schedule the same?

Barriers often appear that prevent the patient from completing the task as originally scheduled. Mental flexibility (discussed in the previous chapter) will allow the patient to generate multiple ways to complete the steps and, ultimately, the total plan.

"Execute" Phase:
How will I know when I'm finished?

Many tasks, like this example, have clear end points: the package is bought, wrapped, and ready to be presented to Bob. Once all the steps of the target task have been identified, sequenced, worked through, and checked off, it is easy to determine the stop point. Other target tasks are more nebulous. For example, how do you know when you have studied enough or when you have saved enough money? Quantifying steps and components for every task will assist the patient in making the determination that it is time to stop.

"Repair" Phase:
What would I do differently? What would I do the same?

If a plan was successful, ask the patient to analyze why it worked so well. Was it that enough time was allowed? Was it that steps were combined in order to make the patient more efficient? Encourage the patient to utilize positive feedback from others and work to incorporate that feedback into future plans. For example, if the birthday card was especially fitting, return to the store and buy a few more for future occasions. Conversely, assist the patient to avoid making the same mistake twice. Determine what did not go well and make alterations to the plan for future use. For example, Bob's birthday occurs at the same time every year. Work toward not scheduling car maintenance at this time next year.

The repair phase needs to be conducted both at the end of the task and throughout the activity.

Planning Form

Task: Have Bob's birthday gift ready by Saturday evening.

Steps	Completion Schedule	✔	Feedback
Balance checkbook. **Need Silence**	15 minutes Sunday afternoon	✔	
Decide budget.	3 minutes Sunday afternoon	✔	
Schedule time to go to the mall.	5 minutes Monday morning	✔	
Schedule time to talk to friends.	with above	✔	
Look in catalogs—check delivery times and fees.	15 minutes Monday evening		Bob said he has trouble with returns not in town—don't use catalogs.
Look online—check delivery times and fees. **Set alarm to limit to 30 minutes.**	30 minutes Monday evening	✔	Got off task looking at other items not related to gift—consider less than 30 minutes and use a louder alarm.
Talk to friends about ideas.	20 minutes Wed. afternoon	✔	
Schedule time to go to the bank.	with third item Monday morning	✔	
Go to the bank.	20 minutes Leave Fri. 5:00pm		
Drive to the store and park.	10 minutes Friday		
Shop and check out—ask for a box. Buy wrap and ribbon. **Keep list handy to stay on track.**	30 minutes Friday		
Drive home.	10 minutes Fri. 8:00pm		
Wrap gift.	10 minutes Sat. 3:00 pm		

Helpful Hints:
- Even as adults, there is something intrinsically satisfying about checking an item off a to-do list. It additionally provides an easy visual summary monitoring completion of the task.

- Checklists are great time savers. Keep these blueprints handy for any repeated task. There is no need to reinvent the wheel each time.

164

Copyright © 2003 LinguiSystems, Inc.

As the patient becomes successful with developing plans, incorporate the development of these plans and the review of plans into the daily planning periods of the daily schedule. Patients should review upcoming or ongoing target projects and their steps daily, and assign them to available time slots within the day or week. The patient's daily to-do list should consist of component steps for many longer term target projects.

Planning Form

Task:

Steps	Completion Schedule	✔	Feedback

Task Steps Activities

Step 1: Check off each item that is critical to the target task.

❏ Wash the sheets.
❏ Strip the bed.
❏ Buy soda at the store.
❏ Call Mary.
❏ Go to the bank.
❏ Buy laundry detergent and fabric softener.
❏ Vacuum the bedroom.
❏ Dry the sheets.
❏ Fluff the pillows.
❏ Find quarters.
❏ Bring the newspaper.
❏ Schedule 1½ hours free.
❏ Collect the dry cleaning.
❏ Drive to the laundromat.
❏ Put the sheets back on the bed.

Step 2: Identify the steps that are omitted from the target task.

✔ Wash the sheets.
✔ Go to the bank.
✔ Buy laundry detergent and fabric softener.
✔ Fluff the pillows.
✔ Find quarters.
✔ Schedule 1½ hours free.
✔ Put the sheets back on the bed.

✔ _____
✔ _____
✔ _____
✔ _____
✔ _____
✔ _____

Task Steps Activities

Step 3:   Write 10 steps you need to take in order to complete the target task.

1. _____

_____

2. _____

_____

3. _____

_____

4. _____

_____

5. _____

_____

6. _____

_____

7. _____

_____

8. _____

_____

9. _____

_____

10. _____

_____

Task Steps Activities

Target: Having the oil in the car changed

Step 1: Check off each item that is critical to the target task.

❑ Clean out the trunk.
❑ Schedule 1 hour free.
❑ Make an appointment.
❑ Replace windshield wiper fluid.
❑ Wash the car.
❑ Drive to the location.
❑ Call Jim.
❑ Have an activity to do while waiting.
❑ Pay car insurance bill.
❑ Pay the bill for the oil change.
❑ Go to the bank.
❑ Drive back home.
❑ Make a notation in the calendar for 3 months later.

Step 2: Identify the steps that are omitted from the target task.

✔ Make an appointment.
✔ Drive to the location.
✔ Have an activity to do while waiting.
✔ Go to the bank.
✔ Make notation in the calendar for 3 months later.

✔ _____

✔ _____

✔ _____

✔ _____

✔ _____

✔ _____

Task Steps Activities

Target: Having the oil in the car changed

Step 3:   Write 10 steps you need to take in order to complete the target task.

1. _____
   _____

2. _____
   _____

3. _____
   _____

4. _____
   _____

5. _____
   _____

6. _____
   _____

7. _____
   _____

8. _____
   _____

9. _____
   _____

10. _____
    _____

Task Sequencing Activities

Ask the patient to answer these questions in order to practice task sequencing.

What are 15 steps involved in brushing your teeth?
1. Turn on the water.
2. Take out the toothbrush.
3. Take out the toothpaste.
4. Unscrew the toothpaste cap.
5. Apply toothpaste to the brush.
6. Wet the toothbrush.
7. Turn off the water.
8. Brush teeth.
9. Turn on the water.
10. Fill a cup with water.
11. Turn off the water.
12. Rinse.
13. Put away the toothbrush.
14. Screw on the toothpaste cap.
15. Put away the toothpaste.

What are 6 steps involved in making a cup of coffee?
1. Determine the number of cups desired.
2. Fill the coffee pot with the appropriate amount of water.
3. Pour the water into the coffee pot.
4. Put a new filter in the coffee grounds basket.
5. Measure the needed number of scoops of coffee into the basket.
6. Turn on the coffee pot.

What are the steps involved in making a bowl of cereal?
1. Take out a bowl.
2. Take out the cereal and open it.
3. Pour the cereal into the bowl.
4. Put the cereal back in the cupboard.
5. Open the refrigerator.
6. Take out the milk.
7. Pour the milk onto the cereal.
8. Put the milk back in the refrigerator.
9. Get a spoon.

Task Combination Activities

Create a schedule to complete each group of tasks within 30 minutes. Combine tasks when appropriate.

- Make a pot of coffee. (5 minutes)
- Make a bowl of cereal. (2 minutes)
- Read the front section of the newspaper. (10 minutes)
- Shower. (12 minutes)
- Make the bed. (3 minutes)
- Get dressed. (10 minutes)

- Unload the dishwasher. (3 minutes)
- Call a friend. (10 minutes)
- Set the table. (5 minutes)
- Pour drinks. (1 minute)
- Cook a casserole. (25 minutes)

- Listen to the nightly news. (30 minutes)
- Open the mail. (3 minutes)
- Wash the towels. (15 minutes)
- Dry the towels. (15 minutes)
- Stamp letters written earlier. (3 minutes)

- Pay bills. (15 minutes)
- Return phone calls. (10 minutes)
- Sort mail. (3 minutes)
- Sort laundry. (4 minutes)

- Make a grocery list. (3 minutes)
- Decide on a menu. (3 minutes)
- Practice the piano. (15 minutes)
- Water the plants. (5 minutes)
- Make a cup of tea. (5 minutes)

Memory

Reductions in memory are a common complaint of people with executive function disorders. Memory is a very complex system that relies on a multitude of other brain functions. Memory is effective only when all the interrelated processes are functioning correctly.

What patients frequently identify as a memory problem is actually a result of reductions in levels of attention, poor planning, and/or difficulty initiating activities. For example, a patient may describe failing to remember anything about a movie he or she saw last week and feel this is due to a poor memory. In reality, the movie taxed sustained attention beyond the patient's ability.

There are an abundance of theories and terms to describe memory, such as immediate, short-term, long-term, working, sensory, tactile, episodic, semantic, and verbal. While it is important for the therapist to have an understanding of these theories and a framework of operation, memory is a difficult, complex neurological process that needs to be simplified for the patient.

Step 1 of Improving Memory

Step 1 of improving memory involves the patient learning and believing four statements:

1. **"You can't remember what you can't pay attention to."**
   The ability to control for deficits in attention is critical to successful recall. The patient must actively anticipate and manipulate the levels of attention a task requires before the process of memory can be successful. Review the section on Attention (page

75) with the patient as it relates to specific items he or she is having difficulty recalling.

- Did the event the patient failed to remember occur after the time limit of his or her sustained attention?
- Did the event take place in a noisy room or with other competing stimuli?
- Was the patient doing something else at the time the event took place?

For example, the patient reports failing to return a call to the plumber who had left a message wishing to change appointment times. Upon query, the patient was listening to the phone messages immediately upon coming in the door. The patient was tired, hungry, and sorting the mail at the same time he was listening to the phone message. This is not a failure to remember as much as a failure in the patient's divided and selective attention. He could not remember what he had not paid attention to. Had the patient listened to the phone messages in isolation with a pen and paper in hand, he would have called the plumber.

2. **"You can't remember what you don't understand."**
New information is more easily recalled when it fits into an existing schema. Conversely, information that cannot fit into a present framework is difficult to process. Understanding the information means not only understanding the words and the meaning, but also how the information fits into the patient's life, organization, and schedule. For example, not attending to or being aware of the plumber's appointment in the first place makes a change in schedule difficult to process and, therefore, difficult to remember.

3. **"You must practice your memory at times when the outcome does not matter — just like you need to practice the piano piece at a time other than at the recital."**
During clinical sessions and as homework, challenge the patient to work on recall for the pure aerobic activity of remembering. Outside of formal education, everyday information tends to be less clearly structured and, therefore, requires more internal manipulation and clarification to be successfully recalled. Patients need to "study" memory and practice methods of recall outside the boundaries of essential tasks.

4. **"Memory is an active process: you must consciously manipulate the information to get it into your head."**
Memory is not a passive process. Information is not stored magically. As adults, however, the processes of storage and retrieval are so overlearned and automatic, they often appear involuntary. Patients frequently state, "I didn't have to do anything to remember before." In fact, their brains did plenty, but patients were not cognizant of the processes working to create a memory.

Step 2 of Improving Memory

The second step of improving memory is to instruct the patient in active methods of storing and retrieving information. The **Memory Techniques** handout on page 180 provides several approaches to improving memory skills. The patient needs to be knowledgeable of the techniques and should be skilled with each.

| **Helpful Hint:** | Ultimately, all components of attention and memory must work cohesively. Manipulate the patient's levels of attention within the clinical memory tasks. |

Memory Techniques

➤ *Repetition:* This includes repeating something over and over in your head. This can be short term, like repeating a phone number received from information just long enough to dial it. If the line is busy when you dial, however, you will probably forget the number. Repetition can also be used for a longer term. By reviewing something day after day after day, it will eventually be stored.

Clinical Practice:
- State and describe the 5 Memory Techniques every session.
- State and describe the 5 types of Attention every session.
- Repeat key sayings in every session, such as., "Plan–Execute–Repair" and "You can't remember what you don't pay attention to."
- Ask the patient to look at the daily schedule at least 3 times per day.
- Ask the patient to look at the daily to-do list at least 3 times per day.
- Ask the patient to look at the target tasks and component steps to particular tasks every day.

➤ *Visualization:* See it in your mind. In a perfect form, visualization is photographic memory. Most of us can't visualize to that level, but perhaps we can recall the color of the book or which side of the page the needed material was on. The same skill can be used to remember if the word is long or short, the graph up or down, etc. We can also visualize by turning information into visual stories, much like a mental videotape, then replaying the "video."

175

Copyright © 2003 LinguiSystems, Inc.

Clinical Practice:
- Provide an assortment of items for the patient to look at for 1 minute. Take the items away and ask the patient to list the items he or she sees. Manipulate the following variables:
  - ✔ the length of presentation time
  - ✔ the number of items presented
  - ✔ the similarity of items
  - ✔ the delay between stimuli and recall

- Ask the patient to gaze at a magazine or newspaper page. Note the visual situation of the page, such as color vs. no color, presence and location of pictures, and number of headlines. Manipulate these variables:
  - ✔ the length of presentation time
  - ✔ the visual complexity of the page
  - ✔ the delay between stimuli and recall

- Ask the patient to describe or draw a room he or she was previously in, such as the waiting room. Manipulate these variables:
  - ✔ the forewarning of the activity
  - ✔ the complexity of the situation
  - ✔ the frequency the situation is encountered
  - ✔ the delay between stimuli and recall

- Ask the patient to provide a description of a person he or she encountered, such as the receptionist. Manipulate these variables:
  - ✔ the forewarning of the activity
  - ✔ the complexity of the situation
  - ✔ the frequency the situation is encountered
  - ✔ the delay between stimuli and recall

- Have the patient read a news story or you read one to the patient. Ask the patient to create a visual image of the actions and people involved. Manipulate these variables:
  - ✔ the forewarning of the activity
  - ✔ the complexity of the story
  - ✔ the familiarity of the story
  - ✔ the length of the story
  - ✔ the delay between stimuli and recall

Copyright © 2003 LinguiSystems, Inc.

➤ *Association:* Tie what the patient is to remember into something he or she already remembers. Build upon previously known facts. Mnemonics are an excellent association tool. "My Very Educated Mother Just Served Us Nine Pies" is a mnemonic to remember the planets. (The beginning letter of each word corresponds to the beginning letter of each planet in the solar system from Mercury outward). The more bizarre the mnemonic, the more inclined your patient will be to recall it.

Clinical Practice:
- Provide the patient with functional word lists, such as grocery items. Help the patient to develop a mnemonic for the list and use this for later recall. Manipulate these variables:
  ✔ the number of words to be recalled
  ✔ the predetermined pattern to the words
     banana, **a**pple, **l**emon, **l**ime = **ball**
  ✔ the delay between stimuli and recall

- Read to the patient or have him or her read a news story about an area of particular interest. Ask the patient to tie the facts into previously known information.

➤ *Grouping:* Place like items together. Know how many items the patient needs to remember and how many groups of items exist. It is challenging to remember 21 grocery items, but it's not difficult to remember 7 meats, 7 vegetables and 7 fruits.

Clinical Practice:
- Provide the patient with a number of items, pictures, or words. Ask the patient to group them into meaningful categories. Manipulate these variables:
  ✔ the number of items
  ✔ the similarity of the items
  ✔ the delay between stimuli and recall

➤ *Write it down:* This is the best method, because if memory fails there is an opportunity to go back and look. The physical act of writing itself is a memory aid.

Clinical Practice:
- Have the patient write notes from a story he or she read or heard. Take the notes away and then ask the patient to recall key facts. Manipulate these variables:
  ✔ the length of the story
  ✔ the interest level of the story
  ✔ the complexity of the story
  ✔ the familiarity of the story
  ✔ the delay between stimuli and recall

- Have the patient take notes on a factual phone call, such as calling to get information about a movie.
- Have the patient take notes on a conversational phone call with a friend.
- Have the patient take notes on a segment from a news program on TV or radio.

Helpful Hint: Always ask the patient how he or she was able to remember something to reinforce the act of active processing. Understanding how memory works is as equally important as answering the questions correctly.

Those people with superior memories can use a variety of techniques simultaneously. Assist the patient in learning which techniques are best for particular situations in daily life.

Clinical Memory Tasks

The **Memory Tasks** on pages 181-183 provide your client with simple word recall activities. Show the patient a grid of 10 words for 2 minutes. Then cover the target words and ask the patient to identify them in the midst of 10 additional words. Here's an example:

Words to memorize:

COMPUTER	HOLIDAY	BALLPARK	MOTORCYCLE
HAMBURGER	TELEVISION	NEWSPAPER	BIRTHDAY
	STADIUM	BICYCLE	

Circle the words previously seen:

LAUNDRY	POLISH	~~BALLPARK~~	~~BICYCLE~~
TORNADO	~~COMPUTER~~	CABINET	~~HOLIDAY~~
NOTEBOOK	~~MOTORCYCLE~~	LAWNMOWER	~~HAMBURGER~~
FIREPLACE	~~TELEVISION~~	TABLECLOTH	OVERCOAT
~~NEWSPAPER~~	~~BIRTHDAY~~	~~STADIUM~~	REFRIGERATOR

Manipulate the difficulty of this task by the following:
- Increase the number of words to be recalled.
- Decrease the time allowed to study.
- Decrease the semantic association of the target words.
- Decrease the visual association of the target words.
- Increase the semantic association of the foil words.
- Increase the visual association of the foil words.
- Ask the patient to recall the target words without cues.
- Decrease the number of words.
- Increase the time allowed to study.
- Increase the semantic association of the target words.

Copyright © 2003 LinguiSystems, Inc.

- Increase the visual association of the target words.
- Decrease the semantic association of the foil words.
  - Increase the visual association of the foil words.
  - Provide the patient with direct cues about which strategy to use and how.

Prospective Memory Tasks

The ability to recall what is to be done in the future is known as **Prospective Memory**. Remembering that a dentist appointment is scheduled next month, that you are supposed to call your accountant next week, or that it is your turn to host Thanksgiving dinner are all examples of prospective memory.

Within the session, require the patient to perform an act in the future, such as one of the following:
- Ask what time the next appointment is scheduled at the end of the session.
- Put a magazine in the waiting room when the session is finished.
- Ask to borrow a pen in 5 minutes or turn off the lights in 10 minutes.
- Write a note about a favorite restaurant to be presented next session.
- Walk to the door in 5 minutes.
- Ask for a glass of water before starting the next session.

Conclusion

There are a variety of compensations for reduced memory. Introduce these compensations as they are appropriate to specific tasks with which the patient is involved:
- Establish set locations for personal items, such as keys, wallets, purses, and cell phones.
- Write a checklist for running errands or doing shopping.
- Use a dictaphone or digital memo recorder to leave yourself messages and notes quickly and easily.
- Have a pencil and paper handy at all times to make notes to yourself.
- Leave yourself reminder messages on your own voice mail.
- Use a tickler file with a folder for each month and a folder for every day. Put birthday cards, invitations and follow-up calls in the folder for the appropriate day and month. Schedule a time to look in these folders daily.

Helpful Hint: Continually check the library and bookstore for publications on improving memory and take notes on strategies suggested in them. Keep your own file of helpful memory tricks to use with patients.

Memory Techniques

Repetition: This includes repeating something over and over in your head. It can be short term, like repeating a phone number you receive from information just long enough to dial. But if the line is busy, you likely will have forgotten the number. Repetition can also be used for a longer term. By reviewing something day after day after day, it will eventually get into your head. By looking at and reviewing the steps involved in completing a task every day, you will remember it.

Visualization: See it in your mind. In a perfect form, visualization is photographic memory. Most of us can't visualize to that level, but perhaps we can recall the color of the book or which side of the page the needed material was on. You can use this same skill to remember if the word is long or short, the graph is up or down, etc. We can also visualize by turning information into stories in our heads, much like a videotape. Then later we can replay the "video."

Association: Tie what you want to remember into something you already remember. Build upon previously known facts. Mnemonics are an excellent association task. "My Very Educated Mother Just Served Us Nine Pies" is a mnemonic to remember the planets. (The beginning letter of each word corresponds to the beginning letter of each planet in the solar system from Mercury outward). The more bizarre the mnemonic, the more inclined you will be to recall it.

Grouping: Place like items together. Know how many things you need to remember and how many groups of items there are. It's challenging to remember 21 grocery items, but it's not difficult to remember 7 meats, 7 vegetables, and 7 fruits.

Write It Down: This is the best method, because if your memory fails you have an opportunity to go back and look at what you wrote. The physical act of writing itself is a memory aid.

 Copyright © 2003 LinguiSystems, Inc.

Memory Tasks

Words to memorize:

DOG	LION	MONKEY	BIRD	FISH
COW	PIG	SNAKE	CAT	HORSE

Circle the words previously seen:

TABLE	FISH	LEAF	WIND	DOG
COW	SHOES	PIG	YELLOW	HORSE
BASKET	LION	SNAKE	DOOR	BIRD
GARAGE	MONKEY	RADIO	CAT	PENCIL

Circle the words previously seen:

TIGER	DOG	COW	GOAT	RABBIT
PIG	LION	BEAR	SPIDER	SQUIRREL
SKUNK	MONKEY	SNAKE	HAMSTER	CAT
RACCOON	BIRD	DONKEY	HORSE	FISH

Words to memorize:

SEED	SUN	SIMPLE	SUGAR	SAID
SOFT	SAME	SAT	SURPRISE	SUPPER

Circle the words previously seen:

HANG	WEST	SAT	LIFT	SAID
SOFT	BLOCK	LOST	SUPPER	SEED
TRUNK	SUN	SIMPLE	JUICE	FRUIT
SAME	SUGAR	BOWL	SURPRISE	LADDER

Circle the words previously seen:

SUPPER	STRAP	STOP	SEED	SHUT
SHOE	SOFT	SUN	SKUNK	SPRING
SAME	STRAW	SUGAR	SPADE	SURPRISE
STEP	SAT	SAID	SCALE	SIMPLE

Memory Tasks

Words to memorize:

COMPUTER	HOLIDAY	BALLPARK	MOTORCYCLE	HAMBURGER
TELEVISION	NEWSPAPER	BIRTHDAY	STADIUM	BICYCLE

Circle the words previously seen:

LAUNDRY	POLISH	BALLPARK	BICYCLE	TORNADO
COMPUTER	CABINET	HOLIDAY	NOTEBOOK	MOTORCYCLE
LAWNMOWER	HAMBURGER	FIREPLACE	TELEVISION	TABLECLOTH
OVERCOAT	NEWSPAPER	BIRTHDAY	STADIUM	CUBE

Words to memorize:

JUMP	LAUGH	SLEEP	EAT	DRIVE
CLEAN	WORK	SPEAK	WATCH	READ
WASH	CHANGE	BLOW	ROLL	FIX
MOVE	PAY	COLLECT	FASTEN	GIVE

Circle the words previously seen:

WORK	BELOW	GIVE	FIX	RECIPE
OTHER	FASTEN	CUP	ROLL	COLLECT
KETTLE	EGGS	BLOW	LAKE	PAY
BIRD	ISLAND	CHANGE	WATCH	MOVE
LIBRARY	WASH	CLEAN	CLOTHES	CLASS
JUMP	LAUGH	WIND	SLEEP	CITY
EAT	SPEAK	DRIVE	BOOK	READ

 Copyright © 2003 LinguiSystems, Inc.

Memory Tasks

Words to memorize:

ORANGE	APPLE	BANANA	LEMON	CHERRY

Circle the words previously seen:

CHAIR	TABLE	LEMON	CHERRY	LAMP
ORANGE	WINDOW	RUG	BANANA	APPLE

Circle the words previously seen:

BEANS	PEAS	APPLE	ORANGE	BROCCOLI
LEMON	CUCUMBER	BANANA	LETTUCE	CHERRY

Documentation

The purpose of documentation is to objectively chart the patient's performance, enabling modifications, as needed, to particular treatment tasks and to the overall goals. It additionally performs a significant role in reimbursement and in providing credibility to both the field and the therapist personally.

Each treatment task must be clearly defined in terms of its functional application. This is not only for the purposes of documentation, but also for allowing the patient a clear understanding of the purpose of any activity. Stating that the patient achieved a particular accuracy in crossing out the letter *M* for 4 lines of small print provides no insight into why that task was selected. People in everyday life are not typically required to cross out letters in 4 lines of small print. More appropriately, this activity would be reported as a selective attention task requiring paper and pencil activity for 1 minute.

Once the task performed has been established in functional terms, the patient's level of performance is stated. Consistent criteria for acceptable vs. unacceptable responses must be established, and there must be a predetermined acceptability standard. To accurately judge performance, the criteria must be invariable and apparent to both the therapist and the patient. Consider the following:

➤ How accurately was each task completed?

➤ How fast/slow were the tasks completed?

➤ How did the speed of performance fluctuate with particular tasks or as the number of cycles increased?

➤ How many breaks were required?

➤ How easy was it to pick up where the patient left off?

➤ How mentally taxing did the patient find the tasks?

➤ Were compensatory strategies used spontaneously?

➤ Were errors identified?

➤ Were errors corrected?

It is not sufficient to simply identify that an error occurred. Identifying *why* that error occurred is imperative. State what area of deficit caused the patient to fail to meet the acceptable criteria. Here is an example:

Reductions in sustained attention caused the patient to be unable to attend to the task for the full 1 minute.

Inability to accurately estimate the time required for the activity caused the patient to be 2 hours off in scheduling 5 daily activities.

Clearly document what you did to modify the task or enhance the patient's performance. State what types of cues you provided, how frequently you provided them, and what effect the cues had on achievement:

The therapist provided an initial verbal cue.

When provided with written cues throughout the task, the patient's total improved to 85%.

The type, frequency, and quantity of the cues you provided to the patient must be established in a consistent manner and documented as such. Cues are typically visual, verbal, tactile, or nonverbal. Additionally, they can be described as follows:

Maximum:	The most direct instruction on how to do the task. The therapist actually shows the patient how to do the task and walks the patient through each step.
Moderate:	The therapist provides cues for greater than 50% of the task.
Modest:	The therapist provides cues for less than 25%-50% of the task.
Minimal:	The least amount of cues provided. Cues may be entirely nonverbal, such as a pause to give the patient time to realize an error. An initial cue at the beginning of the task without further cueing would be minimal.
Independent:	The patient requires no cues from others to complete the task.

The overall performance of a treatment task can be reported using the same 7-point scale employed by the patient to self-assess:

7 = The task was completed accurately and independently.

6 = The task was completed accurately with minimal cues.

5 = Over half of the task was completed accurately and independently.

4 = Over half of the task was completed accurately, given cues.

3 = Less than half of the task was completed accurately and independently.

2 = Less than half of the activity was completed accurately, given cues.

1 = The task was not completed accurately, even with cues.

Stating the functional implications of each treatment activity, clearly defining the acceptable level of performance, evaluating each response in a consistent manner, stating the patient's strengths and weaknesses with the task, and stating the interventions you provided will provide strong documentation.

Sample Treatment Sessions

(Examples for all treatment areas are modeled in these samples of documentation; however, all are not typically accomplished in a characteristic 1-hour session.)

#1 Early in Treatment

1. **Organizational System (Level 2–3)**
   - Does the patient have the organizational system with her?
   - What percent of the time has she carried it since last session?
   - How many appointments/obligations were written into the system this period?
     - Did the patient fail to write any in? Why? How did she come to realize this?
   - Did the patient participate in the **Time Estimation Worksheet**?
   - What percent of activities were estimated within 5 minutes? Overestimated? Underestimated? Discuss.
   - Specific work on time estimation:
     - Patient will estimate within 1 minute how long a newspaper article of interest will take to read (6-8 paragraphs).
     - Patient will estimate within 1 minute how long it will take to travel to the cafeteria.

2. **Attention (Sustained Attention Level)**
   - Restate the 5 types of attention.
   - Can the patient provide examples of when she used each type in her life?
   - Did the patient participate in the **Activity Worksheet**? Discuss.
   - Did the patient report instances of losing sustained attention to a task?
   - What percent of today's situations requiring sustained attention can the patient identify?
   - Has the patient identified time limits and breaks for these tasks?
   - What percent of upcoming situations can the patient identify as taxing sustained attention?
   - Specific practice with sustained attention:
     - Patient will read an article of interest for 2 minutes, take a break, and read for 2 more minutes.
     - Patient will read an article of little interest for 1 minute, take a break, and read for 1 more minute.
     - Patient will visually scan for 1 target letter in medium-sized print for 2 minutes
     - Patient will identify 1 target word from an auditory listing for 1 minute.

3. Memory
➤ Review the 5 techniques to improve memory.
➤ Can the patient provide examples of when each type of memory would be appropriate in her life?
➤ Did the patient experience any specific memory problems during this period? Brainstorm.
➤ Anticipate memory challenges in the upcoming week's events — cues provided.
➤ Specific practice on visualizing:
  • Provide 8 related items for 1 minute of visual examination.
  • Provide 5 unrelated items for 1 minute of visual examination.
  • Play *Concentration* card game with 16 cards.

4. Plan—Execute—Repair
➤ Using a newly-scheduled event on the patient's schedule, can she identify one half of the steps involved in completion of the target task?
➤ With cues, can the patient identify all the steps needed?
➤ With cues, can the patient identify the sequence of the steps?
➤ Specific work on planning:
  • Given a simple map, can the patient get from point A to point B?
  • Can she develop an alternative plan with constraints imposed, such as "no highways"?
  • Sequence 10 steps in a functional task familiar to the patient.
  • Sequence 10 steps in a novel task.

#1 Progress Note

Ms. P brought her organizational system to treatment without a prompt. She reported inconsistent ability to keep it with her throughout the day, particularly when running errands, estimating less than 50% compliance. She reported failing to schedule 1 of 5 appointments this period secondary to not having her system with her and failing to recall to enter the information later on. She recognized the error when she received a reminder call the day before the event. She consistently participated in the Time Estimation Worksheet, entering over 20 events. Ms. P consistently underestimated the time involved in task completion, on one occasion up to 1 hour. She readily agreed that this is an area of difficulty for her and she will continue with the Time Estimation Worksheet during this next period. In specific drill activity, Ms P was 3 minutes off in her estimation of how long a 6-paragraph newspaper article of interest would take to read. She had anticipated that she would be fully accurate in this task. Additionally, she was 2 minutes under in estimating how long it would take to travel to the cafeteria. Again, she anticipated accuracy with this task.

When given an initial verbal cue, the patient was able to state and define all 5 levels of attention. She was 50% accurate stating what types of attention were required for activities from her day. Ms. P reported greater ease in identifying when her sustained attention was faltering but was unable to independently refocus her attention. She participated in the sustained attention analysis but was inaccurate estimating how long she could concentrate on a given task in over half the cases.

On specific drills for sustained attention, she was able to read an article of interest for 2 minutes, break, and then read for 2 more minutes when auditory cues were provided for the break time. She had anticipated success with this task. When given an article of little interest to her, she was able to read for 1 minute, break, and then read for 1 more minute on 1 of 2 attempts when cues for the break were provided. She anticipated being able to complete more than half this task accurately and independently. She was able to maintain her visual attention to a paper and pencil task for 2 minutes but generated 15 errors of omission out of 40. With an auditory task, she maintained her attention for 2 minutes with 5 errors out of 40. She had predicted that she would be able to complete both of these tasks accurately with minimal cues.

The 5 techniques to improve memory were reviewed, with the patient requiring direct cues from the therapist to provide functional examples of their use. Ms. P described daily instances during the previous week where she failed to recall something but was unable to identify why. Direct cues by the therapist assisted her in this realization. Errors were most often the result of failing to write down scheduled events and failure to review the schedule. Specific practice with the compensation of visualization found the patient to recall 6 of 8 similar items presented visually for 1 minute. She was able to recall 2 of 5 unrelated items. Initially, the patient clearly lost sustained attention to the task but did not independently identify this. After a 1-minute break was offered, she returned to the task with the previously-mentioned levels of performance. The patient had predicted that she would complete less than half of this activity accurately, given cues.

When a newly-scheduled event on the patient's schedule was utilized, she was able to independently identify less than half the steps involved in completion. When an array of possible steps was provided, she was able to identify all the steps needed. Once the steps were established, she was able to successfully sequence the steps. With specific work on planning, the patient was able to design a route from point A to point B on a map. She was unable, however, to develop an alternate plan when the constraint of "no highways" was imposed. It required direct visual and verbal cues for the patient to see 2 alternate patterns. She had predicted that she would be able to complete over half of the activity, given cues. When asked to sequence 10 steps in a functional task familiar to her, she was completely accurate. When an unfamiliar task was introduced, however, she was able to sequence only 4 of 10 steps. She had predicted that she could complete this accurately with minimal cues.

Sample Treatment Sessions

#2 Mid–Level in Treatment

1. **Organizational System (Level 7)**
   ➤ Does the patient have the organizational system with her?
   ➤ What percent of the time has she carried it since last session?
   ➤ With what frequency did the patient check her schedule 3 times/day?
   ➤ Did the patient miss any appointments/obligations? Why?
   ➤ Were priorities set daily? If not, why? Follow up.
   ➤ What problems in time management were encountered this last period? Brainstorm.

2. **Attention (Selective Attention Level)**
   ➤ Restate the 5 types of attention.
   ➤ Can the patient provide examples of when she used each type in her life?
   ➤ Does the patient report any difficulties with sustained attention this period?
   ➤ What percent of situations from the last period requiring selective attention can the patient identify?
   ➤ How did the patient manage these situations?
   ➤ Direct practice on selective attention:
     • Patient reads 3 paragraphs with quiet music in the background.
     • Patient attempts moderate level word retrieval activities in the gym.

3. **Memory**
   ➤ Review the 5 techniques to improve memory.
   ➤ Can the patient provide examples of when each type would be appropriate in her life?
   ➤ Did the patient experience any specific memory problems this period? Brainstorm.
   ➤ Anticipate memory challenges in the upcoming week's events (cues provided).
   ➤ Specific practice on grouping:
     • Provide 20 words with 2 obvious groupings.
     • Provide 10 words with less obvious groupings.

191

Copyright © 2003 LinguiSystems, Inc.

4. Plan—Execute—Repair
➤ Review the patient's currently established plans:
- Did the patient perform all scheduled tasks? Why or why not?
- Did the patient participate in the repair phase with these tasks?

➤ Are there newly-scheduled tasks requiring a plan?
- Did the patient independently instigate attempts to generate a plan? Provide cues.

➤ Specific work on planning:
- Identify 3 available time options for treatment next week.
- Identify pros and cons of each time option.
- Identify the time frame for homework activities to be completed prior to the night before.

#2 Progress Note

Ms. P brought her organizational system to treatment without a prompt. She reported consistent, independent ability to keep it with her throughout the day. She reported being late for 1 of 4 scheduled appointments this period secondary to inaccurately anticipating the travel time involved. She consistently identified 1-2 priority activities each day given cues by the therapist. She completed 3 of 5 priority items — on 2 occasions she failed to check her schedule until after the opportunity passed. On the other occasion, another task developed that she felt was more important. The original priority item was independently rescheduled.

The patient was able to independently state and define all 5 levels of attention. She was 75% accurate stating what types of attention were required for activities from her day. Ms. P reported easily maintaining her attention to a variety of tasks for up to 10 minutes, independently utilizing compensatory strategies. In direct practice of selective attention, she was 80% accurate answering questions about a 4-paragraph news article of interest that she read while inhibiting a quiet auditory stimuli. She was 60% accurate in moderate-level word retrieval tasks in the midst of moderate visual and auditory stimuli. She had predicted that she would be able to complete both of these tasks accurately with minimal cues. Her lower performance in the word retrieval task was surprising to her as she did not think the presence of noise and action would distract her from the task.

The 5 techniques to improve memory were reviewed, with the patient requiring direct cues from the therapist to provide functional examples of their use. Ms. P described 3 instances during the previous week where she failed to recall something. For 2 of these instances she independently analyzed the difficulty but required cues to determine strategies for compensation.

192

Copyright © 2003 LinguiSystems, Inc.

Specific practice with the compensation of grouping found the patient to recall 15 of 20 random items falling into 2 pre-established categories. She was able to recall 5 of 10 items when no groupings were provided. The patient had predicted that she would complete less than half of this activity accurately given cues and was pleased with how many items she was able to recall.

The patient had with her the 2 established plans for executing 2 ongoing activities. She successfully performed all the scheduled tasks during this period. She had not, however, analyzed the success or failure of these tasks and required direct cues to determine what aspects should be modified in the future. The patient identified 1 additional activity that would require the development of a plan; however, she had made no attempts to begin this plan. Once cued to do so, she was able to independently identify 5 steps and their sequence.

In specific work on planning, she required direct cues from the therapist to determine 3 available time options for the next treatment session. She was unable to determine possible rearrangements to her schedule when an alternate time was suggested. The patient had predicted she would complete this activity accurately and independently. She did not recognize the difficulty she had when her planned schedule was not accepted and needed alteration.

Copyright © 2003 LinguiSystems, Inc.

Sample Treatment Sessions

#3 Nearing the End of Treatment

1. Organizational System (Level 11)
- ➤ Does the patient have the organizational system with her?
- ➤ Does she continue to be consistent in carrying it with her at all times?
- ➤ Does the patient continue to independently check her schedule 3 times/day?
- ➤ Did the patient miss any appointments/obligations? Why?
- ➤ Were priorities set daily? If not, why? Follow up.
- ➤ Does the patient continue to be consistent in following routines?
- ➤ Given this week's schedule, was the patient able to identify situations where the schedule or plan may not go as anticipated?
- ➤ In these instances, what percent of the time did the patient identify an alternate plan?
- ➤ In these instances, what percent of the time did the patient identify more than 1 alternate plan?
- ➤ If a change in schedule occurred, was the patient successful in initiating an alternate plan?
- ➤ What problems in time management were encountered this last period? Brainstorm.
- ➤ Specific practice:
  - • Given a scenario, identify 5 possible obstacles to the plan.
  - • Identify 3 possible solutions.

2. Attention (Divided Attention Level)
- ➤ Restate 5 types of attention.
- ➤ Can the patient provide examples of when she used each type in her life?
- ➤ Does the patient report any difficulties with sustained attention this period?
- ➤ Does the patient report any difficulties with selective attention this week?
- ➤ What percent of situations from the last period requiring divided attention can the patient identify?
- ➤ How did the patient manage these situations?
- ➤ Direct practice on divided attention:
  - • Patient reads 3 paragraphs with the weather report in the background, identifying the low temperature for the day.
  - • Patient attempts moderate level word retrieval activities in the gym for 3 minutes while keeping track of how many people use the treadmill.
  - • Patient performs visual scanning of standard print-sized letters, scanning for *s*, *a*, and *h* for 5 minutes.

3. Memory
➤ Review the 5 techniques to improve memory.

➤ Can the patient provide examples of when each type would be appropriate in her life?

➤ Did the patient experience any specific memory problems during this period? Brainstorm.

➤ Anticipate memory challenges in the upcoming week's events (cues provided).

➤ Specific practice on associations:
  • Provide 10 faces and names for the patient to learn and recall (direct cues for method of association).
  • Provide 5 faces and names for the patient to learn and recall without cues.
  • Recall main point and details from the 10-paragraph newspaper article of interest that she read last session.
  • Have patient provide all possible meanings for difficult level homonyms.

4. Plan–Execute–Repair
➤ Review the patient's currently established plans:
  • Are plans in existence for all current tasks?
  • Did the patient perform all scheduled tasks? Why or why not?
  • Did the patient participate in the repair phase with these tasks?
  • What percent of previously-designed plans is the patient reusing?

➤ Did the patient miss any appointments this period?

➤ Was the patient tardy with any deadlines?

➤ Specific work on repair:
  • Given a previously-used plan and different constraints/guidelines, what alterations should she make?

#3 Progress Note

Ms. P brought her organizational system to treatment without a prompt. She reported consistent, independent ability to keep it with her throughout the day. She reported consistent timelines with appointments and obligations this period. She consistently and independently identified 1-2 priority activities each day. She completed 4 of 5 priority items. The missed item was dropped in favor of another task that she felt was more important. The original priority item was independently rescheduled. Ms. P reported consistently following her pre-established routines. When something interfered with the routine, she reported rescheduling approximately 90% of the time. Ms. P was able to anticipate 60% of possible interference with her schedule. With cues from the therapist, this increased to 90%. She was independent in her ability to generate 1 alternative plan, 70% in developing 2 alternatives, and 25% in developing 3 alternatives. Ms. P predicted she would require cues for this but that she would be over half correct.

Copyright © 2003 LinguiSystems, Inc.

The patient was able to independently state and define all 5 levels of attention. She was accurate stating what types of attention were required for activities from her day. Ms. P reported easily maintaining her attention to a variety of tasks for up to 20 minutes, independently utilizing compensatory strategies. She reported continued difficulty maintaining her concentration in noisy environments but reported independent ability to utilize compensatory strategies for this.

In direct practice of divided attention, she was 60% accurate answering questions about a 4-paragraph news article of interest that she read while simultaneously listening to the radio. She was successful in identifying the target auditory stimuli from the radio (low temperature for the day). She was 75% accurate in moderate-level word retrieval tasks in the midst of moderate visual and auditory stimuli. Ms. P was simultaneously able to attend to a target visual stimuli (keeping track of people using the treadmill). She had predicted that she would be able to complete over half of both of these tasks accurately without cues. She was 85% accurate in dividing her attention among 3 target items in a visual scanning task. Again, Ms. P thought she would be able to complete over half of this task accurately without cues.

Ms. P was independent in her ability to state and define 5 techniques to improve memory and to provide functional examples of their use. Ms. P described 1 instance during the previous week where she failed to recall something. She independently identified that she had been distracted by another task at the time the information was presented to her and did not actively utilize any memory strategies. In reviewing her schedule for the week, she was able to identify at least 1 challenge to memory for each of 5 scheduled activities. She required cues to identify an additional challenge. At this point, she was independently able to provide an example of a strategy that would be helpful.

Specific practice with the compensation of association found the patient to recall 7 of 10 random names to match faces when the association method was provided to her. She was able to recall 3 of 5 names when no direction was provided. The patient had predicted that she would complete less than half of this activity accurately given cues and was pleased with how many items she was able to recall. Ms. P was asked to recall the main point from a newspaper article she read 5 days prior and had been instructed to recall. She recalled 50% of the supporting facts independently—100% when cues from the therapist were provided. The patient had predicted that she would be able to do this accurately and without assistance. Ms. P was able to provide 1 additional meaning for difficult level homonyms 100% of the time, 2 meanings 75% of the time, and all possible meanings 45% of the time.

The patient continues to demonstrate success in establishing and carrying out plans. She independently completed all scheduled tasks this week and did not miss or was not late for any appointments or deadlines. She has established set times for routine activities and is independent in their execution. She continues to have difficulty anticipating possible obstacles to her plans. In specific treatment tasks, she was able to generate 1 alternative to her plan when a different constraint was identified by the therapist. She was, however, unable to independently identify possible alterations to the plan. She consistently participates in the Repair Phase of activities and makes written notes on her original plan. She has not, however, utilized previously-established plans and their repair comments for recurring tasks, despite opportunity and cues to do so.

197

Copyright © 2003 LinguiSystems, Inc.

Page 134

big, big little, little, big, little big
big , little, big, little, little, little, little
big, big, little, big, big, little, little
little, big, little ,big, big, little, big
little, little, big, big, little, big, little
little, little, little, big, big, little, big
big, little, little, little, big, big, little
big, big, little, big, little, little, big
big, little, big, little, little, little, little
big, big, little, big, little, big, big
little, big, little, little, little, little, big
big, little, big, little, little, big, big
little, big, little, little, little, little, big
big, little, big, little, big, big, little
big, little, little, big, little, big, big
little, big, little, little, little, little, big
big, little, big, big, little, little, little
little, big, little, big, big, little, big
little, little, big, big, big, big, little
big, little, little, little, little, big, big
big, little, little, little, little, big, big
little, big, little, big, big, big, little
big, little, big, little, little. little, little

Page 135

fat, skinny, skinny, fat, fat
skinny, skinny, fat, skinny, skinny
skinny, fat, fat, fat, skinny
fat, skinny, skinny, skinny, fat
skinny, skinny, fat, fat, skinny
skinny, fat, skinny, skinny, skinny
skinny, fat, skinny, fat, fat
fat, skinny, fat, skinny, skinny
skinny, skinny, skinny, fat
skinny, fat, skinny, fat, skinny
skinny, skinny, skinny, fat, skinny
skinny, skinny, skinny, skinny, skinny
fat, skinny, fat, fat, skinny
skinny, skinny, skinny, skinny, skinny
skinny, fat, fat, skinny, skinny
fat, fat, skinny, fat, skinny
skinny, fat, skinny, skinny, skinny
skinny, skinny, fat, skinny, fat
skinny, skinny, skinny, fat, skinny
fat, fat, skinny, fat, skinny
skinny, skinny, fat, fat, fat
skinny, skinny, fat, skinny, skinny
fat, skinny, skinny, skinny, fat

Page 136

print, print, cursive, print, cursive, cursive
print, cursive, print, cursive, cursive, cursive
print, cursive, print, print, print, cursive
print, print, cursive, cursive, print, print
cursive, cursive, print, print, print, print
cursive, print, print, cursive, print, cursive
print, print, cursive, print, cursive, print
cursive, cursive, cursive, print, print, print
print, print, print, cursive, cursive, cursive
cursive, print, print, print, print, print
print, cursive, cursive, print, cursive, print
cursive, cursive, print, print, print, cursive
print, cursive, print, cursive, print, print
cursive, print, cursive, print, print, cursive
print, print, cursive, cursive, cursive, print
print, cursive, cursive, print, print, cursive
cursive, print, print, cursive, print, print
print, cursive, cursive, print, cursive, print
print, print, cursive, print, print, cursive
print, print, print, cursive, cursive, print
print, print, print, print, print, print
cursive, cursive, cursive, print, print, print
print, cursive, cursive, print, cursive, print

Page 137

bold, bold, light, light, bold, light, bold
bold, bold, light, light, light, bold, light
bold, light, light, bold, light, bold, bold
bold, bold, light, light, bold, light, bold
bold, light, light, bold, light, bold, bold
bold, bold, light, bold, light, light, light
bold, light, bold, light, light, bold, light
bold, bold, bold, bold, light, light, light
bold, light, bold, bold, light, light, bold
light, bold, bold, bold, bold, light, bold
light, light, light, bold, light, bold, bold
bold, light, light, light, bold, light, bold
bold, light, light, bold, light, bold, bold
light, light, bold, light, bold, bold, bold
bold, light, light, bold, light, bold, bold
bold, light, light, light, bold, light, bold
bold, light, bold, light, light, bold, light
bold, bold, bold, bold, light, bold, light
light, light, bold, light, bold, bold, bold
light, light, light, light, bold, bold, bold
bold, light, light, bold, bold, bold, bold
light, bold, light, light, bold, bold, bold

Page 139

97,92,138,133,93,142,128,101,104,116,83,163,153
5,56,39,22,38,0,40,36,56,18,48,6,74
139,119,98,174,165,157,168,148,130,108,122,179,130
72,8,55,11,0,14,5,76,10,38,6,48,24
85,139,88,134,66,129,128,104,172,129,184,166,135
50,46,26,50,41,39,47,42,15,11,31,26,37

Copyright © 2003 LinguiSystems, Inc.

139,106,150,120,101,135,120,165,194,107,132,109,111
27,19,56,30,64,51,32,18,58,50,17,17,35
88,140,137,147,93,97,115,76,147,131,100,140,117
2,37,8,34,64,34,9,64,21,33,36,69,26
172,132,80,139,83,108,116,154,118,116,180,102,127

Page 140
172,62,80,55,83,22,116,34,118,2,180,48,127
7,92,8,53,13,142,26,101,4,116,29,161,23
143,56,31,130,42,54,40,148,34,46,52,184,74,
139,65,98,30,165,13,168,34,130,88,122,17,140
68,178,45,187,0,64,5,102,7,136,6,102,24
85,13,88,18,66,29,125,32,172,69,184,14,135
55,142,14,108,35,117,53,106,25,115,9,142,37
196,14,150,74,101,43,120,9,164,21,132,37,111
33,155,6,166,6764,143,28,156,8,108,37,159,35
88,10,137,50,93,15,95,26,147,19,100,30,117
2,79,8,34,64,90,9,112,21,121,36,117,3

Page 141
139,45,351,174,165,595,9,534,21,120,102,68,33
128,154,90,128,46,116,111,22,162,3,69,118,4
69,35,198,456,80,48,125,42,163,32,588,14,609
316,100,25,54,43,702,348,97,9,9,115,142,498
96,52,344,62,66,268,204,51,588,30,132,216,101
33,19,6,166,480,51,28,156,8,118,27,149,366
184,375,7,88,83,15,414,255,49,19,100,116,612
28,69,39,118,696,90,29,102,22,450,36,117,3,
378,36,66,77,39,329,336,85,7,54,19,248,273
148,162,279,94,76,511,246,96,86,18,92,84,140

Page 146

accident	mishap, by chance, car crash
account	statement of transactions and resulting balance, formal contractual relationship, narrative record of events, statement that explains or gives reasons for an action or event
act	something people do, legal document, part of a play, perform an action, behave in a certain manner, play a role or a part
admit	allow participation, allow to enter, means of entrance, acknowledge actions, have room for
appreciate	increase in value, be fully aware of, to show gratitude for
arm	body part, supply with ammunition
ash	tree, remains of something burned
average	statistic, middle, common
back	position in football, a support, body part, furthest from the front, the side that is not seen, be behind
bail	temporarily release from custody, remove water with a container
ball	pitch not in the strike zone, round toy, formal dance
band	bind or tie together, stripe of contrasting color, group of musicians, circular piece of jewelry
bangs	fringe of hair across forehead, loud noises, vigorous blows, closes violently
bank	building where money transactions occur, sloping land, a supply held in reserve for future use, a container for keeping money at home
bar	counter, act of prevention, a block of solid substance, body of individuals qualified to practice law, rigid piece of wood or metal
bark	sound made by a dog, protective covering of a tree, to speak in unfriendly tones
base	a support or foundation, place a base runner in baseball must touch before scoring, military headquarters, lowest part, principal ingredient in a mixture
baste	sewing stitch, cooking method
bat	a turn swinging in baseball, animal, a club used in hitting a ball, flutter one's eyelashes, to strike violently
batter	a flour mixture, a ballplayer who is batting
beam	long piece of material used in construction, gymnastic apparatus, smile radiantly
bear	animal, optimistic investor, take on as one's own, have rightfully, give birth, bring forth, to put up with
beat	regular rate of repetition, regular route for a police officer, contraction and expansion of the heart, glaring with intensity, to mix, to be superior, to win in competition, hit repeatedly, subject or area covered by a reporter

 Copyright © 2003 LinguiSystems, Inc.

bed	furniture, plot of ground, bottom of ocean
bell	hollow device made of metal that makes a ringing sound, percussion instrument, button on an outer door, grading curve
belt	a band of material to tie or buckle around waist, endless band of material between two pulleys, hit vigorously, sing loudly
bend	curved segment of road or river, movement that causes the formation of curve, to change direction
bill	rim of a hat that shades the eyes, statement of money owed, a statute before it becomes law, part of a bird, to request money
bit	cutting part of a drill, piece of metal held in a horse's mouth by reins, a small fragment, unit of measurement of information, an instance of some kind, an indefinite short period of time, a short performance, injured by teeth or stings
blank	explosive charge without a bullet, a substitute for a taboo word, a surface not written on, a gap or missing part, empty space used to separate words
block	a solid piece of material, an inability to remember or think of something you normally can do, quantity of related things, rectangular area in a city, to prohibit something or someone from moving forward
blow	forceful exhalation, powerful stroke with fist or weapon, an unpleasant surprise, a strong current of air, burst suddenly, spend wastefully
blue	color, feeling sad
bluff	steep bank, to deceive an opponent in a card game
board	flat piece of wood; food or meals; a committee having supervisory powers; a device for controlling other electrical devices; to get on a train, bus, or airplane
boil	a painful sore, to cook in hot water, to be in a state of agitation, to change from liquid to vapor

bolt	sudden abandonment, a type of screw, roll of cloth, a discharge of lightning, secure with a lock, in a rigid manner
bore	hole made by a drill, an uninteresting person
boss	a person responsible for employees, to order people around
bow	a piece used in playing stringed instruments, a knot used with shoelaces, a decorative ribbon
bowl	a round dish, to participate in the game of bowling, an important college football game
box	to hit, a container, separate area in a public place, area on a baseball diamond where the hitter or coach stands, rectangular drawing, to participate in the sport of boxing
brake	car part used to slow or stop a vehicle, to apply pressure to the pedal in a car or on a bike, stroke of luck
brand	a name given to a product or service, identification mark on skin, a symbol of disgrace
brick	rectangular block of clay, a solid block of material
bridge	a card game, structure that allows people or vehicles to cross an obstruction, upper deck of a ship, the link between two lenses, a dental treatment, to connect or reduce the distance between
brief	a condensed written summary, to give essential information to someone, of short duration, type of underwear
buck	male of various animals, one dollar, move quickly and violently
buckle	fastener, to fold or collapse
bug	insect, hidden microphone, a fault or defect, annoy persistently
bump	an impact, a lump on the body, a type of dance, reduce in rank, came upon by accident
cable	strong thick rope, television system, a telegram sent abroad

cabinet	a storage compartment, an advisory body of government
calf	baby cow, fine leather, body part
can	metal container, slang for bathroom, to be able to, expresses permission, to terminate employment
cap	headwear, top of a mushroom, lid, dental application, an upper limit, small explosive used in toy guns
case	portable container, glass container for display, actual state of things, statements of fact, a problem requiring investigation, an occurrence of something, a person requiring services, the outer cover of something, a person of a specified kind, to look over
cast	object formed by a mold, hard bandage, a group of actors in a performance, throwing something, to place a vote, to assign roles to actors, formulate in a particular style or language
center	a position in basketball or ice hockey, a building dedicated to a particular activity, cluster of cells governing a specific bodily process, the object that interest is focused, the middle
change	to put on a different set of clothes, a thing that is different, the result of alteration or modification, an event that happens when something passes from one state or phase to another, money received in return for its equivalent, a group of coins
channel	a television frequency, a path that electrical signals pass over, a means of communication, body of water, to direct the flow of
charge	to rush toward something, request of payment, a person committed to your care, the purchase price charged of an article or service, an assertion that someone is guilty of an offense, to refresh a battery, to pay with credit card
charm	something believed to be good luck, attractiveness, small ornament on a bracelet

check	to inspect something, a maneuver in chess and ice hockey, a textile pattern, the bill in a restaurant, a written order for a bank to pay money, a mark indicating something has been completed, consign for shipment, make an investigation, to verify
chest	box with a lid, furniture with drawers, body part
china	a country, high quality porcelain
chip	electrical equipment, used to represent money in gambling, thin slice of potato, cow excrement, fragment of something broken from the whole, short golf shot
chop	karate term, cut of meat, hit sharply
class	elegance, the same social or economic status, things sharing a common attribute, a group of students that are taught together, body of students who graduate together, a league ranked by quality
clip	fastener, to fasten, a short preview of a presentation, to cut
club	stout stick, playing card symbol, group of people, a building, golf equipment, entertainment spot, to hit something or someone
clutch	car part, a critical situation, to grasp
coat	the fur covering an animal, article of clothing, a thin layer covering something, to cover the surface of something
cold	absence of heat, a mild infection, loss of conscious, feeling or showing no affection or friendliness
colon	body part, punctuation mark
company	an institution created to conduct business, a unit of fire fighters, guests, small military unit, to be a companion to someone
complex	complicated, a psychological disorder or condition, a group of buildings or structures
concentration	strengthening by removing extraneous material, spatial property, complete attention, increase in density

contact	close interaction, touching physically, a person who can give special assistance, to communicate with
corn	vegetable, hard thickening of the skin
count	to list numbers in order, a nobleman, to carry weight, to have faith in, to show consideration for
counter	table with horizontal surface, a return punch, speak in response, indicating opposite, deal with ahead of time
court	area where a game is played, residence of a nobleman, an assembly to conduct judicial business, engage in social activities
cover	blanket, the act of concealing something, be sufficient to meet
crab	a grouch, a crustacean
crack	a brief attempt, an illegal drug, a sudden sharp noise, a long narrow opening, witty remark, to fracture
crane	bird, machinery, to move the neck in order to see better
creep	someone unpleasant, to move slowly, to grow in a way as to cover
cricket	a game, a leaping insect
critical	calling attention to errors and flaws, verging on a state of crisis or emergency, having the nature of a turning point, urgently needed
crop	yield from plants, to have hair cut short
cross	an emblem of Christianity, a marking consisting of crossing lines, mixing breeds of animals, to cover a wide area, meet and pass
curb	edge between sidewalk and road, limiting excess
dampen	make moist, smother or suppress
dart	a tuck make in sewing, sudden quick movement, a game piece
dash	quick run, with great haste, distinctive elegance, part of morse code, a race, punctuation mark, destroy, a small amount in cooking
date	fruit, participant in an outing, an outing, the present, specific day of the year

deal	distributing playing cards, particulars of buying or selling, type of treatment received, an agreement between parties, large amount
deck	platforms on a boat or house, 52 playing cards, knock down with force, decorate
decline	change to something smaller or lower, go down, get worse, to refuse to accept, get smaller
dip	a quick swim, a brief immersion, sauce to dunk bite-sized foods into, a depression in a level surface, to go down momentarily
direction	a general course, a description of how something is done, a line leading to a place or point, managing something
dock	landing in a body of water, a platform for loading and unloading, deduct from wages
down	a play in football, soft fine feathers, eat a lot, not functioning, shut, understood perfectly

page 147

draft	a preliminary sketch, a regulator to control air, a drink, a current of air, a document, compulsory military service, to draw up or outline
draw	a poker play, anything taken at random, the finish of a contest with no winner, to remove blood, represent with a picture
dress	clothing, to put clothes on, to bandage a wound, provide with clothes, prepare for market or consumption, groom with elaborate care
drill	tool, training in marching and use of weapons, learning by repetition
drop	central depository, a sharp decrease in quantity, rapid descent, predetermined hiding place, a small amount of liquid, terminate an association, stop pursuing, utter casually
duck	bird, heavy cotton fabric, to move quickly, avoiding the issue
dull	less lively, boring, not sharp, not keenly felt, made softer or less loud

ear	body part, keen hearing, fruiting spike of corn
egg	animal reproductive body, to throw eggs at someone or something, to goad
elder	person who is older than you, church officer, bush
endorse	signing checks or documents, guarantee, give support
engage	participate, to be married, start, get caught
eye	body part, small hole in needle, good discernment, to look at, middle of a storm
face	confronting bravely, outward appearance of something, front of the head, status in the eye of others
fair	competitive exhibition, light colored, free of clouds or rain, baseball hit between the foul lines, free of favoritism, not excessive
fall	a lapse, movement downwards, sudden decline, a season, lose power or office
fan	device for creating a current of air, ardent follower, strike out a batter in baseball, agitate the air
fast	abstaining from food, permanently dyed, acting or moving quickly, hurried and brief
felt	fabric, detected by instinct, touch
file	tool for smoothing metal or wood, office furniture, set of related records, register in a public office, to smooth
film	thin coating, photographic material, form of entertainment, to record
fine	money charged as a penalty, texture, above average, characterized by elegance, minutely precise, good health, being satisfactory
finish	the end, downfall of someone, decorative surface
fire	shooting weapons, intense criticism, burning event, severe trial, terminate, bake in a kiln, provide with fuel
firm	members of a business, make taut, not likely to fluctuate, not shaky, unwavering, not soft, secure
fit	display of temper, sudden flurry of activity, uncontrollable attack, right size or shape, insert or adjust, be compatible, physically or mentally sound
flag	emblem, stone, signaling device, communicate or signal, draw attention to
flat	deflated tire, shallow seedling box, suite of rooms on one floor, lack of carbonation, not glossy, having no depth, lacking enthusiasm
float	remains on the surface of liquid, time between deposit of check and payment, ice-cream drink, circulate, move lightly
flounder	fish, behave awkwardly, walk with difficulty
flush	sudden rapid flow of water, poker hand, reddening of the face, sensation of heat, cause to flow
fly	insect, opening in pants, lure, quick change of emotions, travel by plane, to be airborne
foil	thin sheet of metal, picture viewed with a projector, hinder or prevent
fool	person lacking judgment, indulge in horseplay, to trick
foot	body part, support resembling a pedal, unit of length, lowest support of a structure, to pay for something, to walk
fork	cutlery, branching out, agricultural tool, split in a road
foul	violation of the rules of a sport, disgustingly dirty, obscenity, outside of a boundary
frame	still photographs on a strip of film, human body, supporting structure, enclosure for a picture, catch in a trap
free	no charge, lack of confinement, lack of obligation, remove obstruction, part with
fret	agitation caused from worry, erode, carve a pattern into, metal bar in a musical instrument
fudge	soft candy, falsify or fake

 Copyright © 2003 LinguiSystems, Inc.

game	a contest, informal term for occupation, animal hunted for food or sport
gear	toothed wheel, equipment for a sport, to set the level
general	a fact about the whole, ranking officer, prevailing among the public, not specific
glasses	eyewear, containers for holding liquid
grade	gradient of a slope or road, degree of value, a number or letter of quality, group of students of the same age
grate	frame to hold a fire, bars blocking passage but admitting air, harsh, scraping sound, reduce to shreds, make resentful
graze	superficial abrasion, break the skin, eat lightly, feed in a pasture
grease	thick fatty oil, lubricate, to apply oil
green	color, grass on a golf course, unhealthy appearance, not ripe, naive, envious
grill	framework of metal bars, restaurant, cooking method, intense questioning
groom	recently married man, horse stable worker, care for appearance, preparing for a future role
ground	connection between an electrical device and the earth, a position to be won, motive, top layer of the earth where plants are grown
gum	tissue surrounding base of teeth, a preparation for chewing, tree, chew without teeth
hail	greeting, precipitation, call for, praise
ham	meat, exaggerate ones actions
hamper	container for clothes, restraint that restricts freedom, put at a disadvantage
hand	physical assistance, body part, pointer on a timepiece, ability, one of two sides to an issue, round of applause, cards held in a card game, ship's crew member
hard	strong, dried out, unfortunate, not yielding to pressure, difficult, with effort
harp	musical instrument, lampshade supports, nag or repeat in an annoying fashion
hatch	moveable barrier, birth from an egg, sit on, devise or invent
haze	reduced visibility, confusion, initiation rituals
head	one side of a coin, body part, top of something, foam on a drink, person in charge, tip of an abscess, difficult juncture, travel towards
hide	body covering of an animal, dressed skin of an animal, prevent from being seen, to conceal
hike	long walk, increase in cost, salary increase
hit	big success, striking something, successful play in sports, dose of a drug, affect suddenly, come in sudden contact, suddenly realize
hood	engine covering, hat connected to coat, exhaust vent, young criminal, slang for neighborhood
host	animal or plant that supports a parasite, bread used in communion, to provide facilities for an event, vast amount, person responsible for guests at an event, emcee
ice	frozen water, diamonds, skating rink, medical treatment
incline	make receptive, tendency to do something, elevated geological formation
iron	home appliance, golf club, branding tool, metal shackles, metallic element, to press clothes
jack	male name, tool, face card, game piece, electronic device
jam	preserve of crushed fruit, crowd, difficult situation, interfere or prevent signals, bruise, get stuck
jar	container, sudden impact, affect in a disagreeable way, shock physically
jerk	spasmodic movement, an annoying person
judge	public official, form an opinion, determine the result of competition

key	metal device for security, pitch of the voice, crucial, a list that explains symbols, tonal frame work for music, vandalize a car
kid	young goat, soft leather, human off-spring, to tease
kind	type, showing consideration
knock	rapping, negative criticism, bad experience, car engine noise
knot	looping and tying, twisted and swollen, navigational unit of measure, tangle or complicate
lace	delicate fabric, cord to fasten shoes, to draw thru eyes or holes, mix with alcohol
land	solid part of the earth, territory occupied by a nation, deliver a blow, come to a rest, arrive on shore
lap	movement once around a course, upper thighs when seated, touching with the tongue
last	the lowest in order, duration, end of life, most unlikely, not to be altered
lean	rely on for support, to incline or bend, have a tendency to do, little excess, lacking fat
leaves	periods away from military service, departing politely, remove from participation, make possibility for, have as a remainder, be survived by, refrain from changing, go away from a place
left	opposite of right, have gone, liberal political orientation, remainder
letter	written message, award for athletic or extracurricular participation, single character of the alphabet, literal interpretation
lie	untruth, manner in which something is situated, a place in relation to something else, to remain in particular state
light	illumination device, visual effect in pictures, public awareness, mental understanding, another perspective, fondly regarded
like	feel about, fond of, find enjoyable, want to have, wish to do something, equal in amounts
limb	arm or leg, tree branch, taking a chance
line	conforming, cord or rope, railroad track, commercial organization, kind of product, conceptual separation, mark that is long relative to its width, text, mark indicating bounds of the playing area
lip	body part, top edge of something
loaf	shaped mass of bread, to be lazy
lock	wrestling hold, fastener to secure something, cluster of hair
lodge	hotel, association of people with similar interests, implant, to provide housing for
log	piece of wood, book for keeping track of events, to keep track of events
long	opposite of short, to miss someone
lounge	a place or room for relaxation, to relax, a type of reclining chair
maroon	purplish color, to leave stranded, isolate without resources
mask	concealing activity, a covering to disguise the face, shield from light
mass	celebration of the eucharist, having weight, collection of similar things, large number, occurring widely
match	coated piece of wood or cardboard used for starting fires, exact duplicate, formal contest, a person of equal standing, provide funds, bring two ideas, people, objects together
mate	officer on a ship, Australian term for *friend*, partner of an animal, chess move, exact duplicate, fellow member of a team, copulate, partner in marriage
mean	specified degree of importance, denotes, intend to express, have a purpose in mind, logical consequence, excellent, unkind
meet	athletic contest, collect in one place, get together socially, satisfy, get to know, come together, undergo

page 148

might	physical strength, express possibility, express permission
milk	dairy beverage, exploit
mine	explosive device, excavation of the earth, possession
mint	plant where money is coined, candy, plant, a lot of something
miss	failure to hit, young woman, be absent, fail to experience, fail to reach, feel the lack of, leave out
mold	container that liquid is poured into to create a shape, fungus, fit tightly, shape or influence
mole	animal, spot on the skin, spy, molecular weight
mug	container with a handle, human face, to rob, to smile broadly at a camera
nail	pointed piece of metal, covering of the tip of a finger or toe, attach something, locate exactly, succeed, take into custody, hit hard
nap	a short sleep, period of time spent sleeping, fuzzy texture
negative	film with black and white tones reversed, denial, number less than zero, unpleasant, disagreeable
novel	fictional work, pleasantly different, of a kind not seen before
nut	small metal block with internal screw thread, large hard seed, someone devoted to something, eccentric person
orange	color, citrus fruit
order	document, body of rules, command, request for food, arrangement of elements, proper arrangement, legal command, association of people with similar interests
organ	wind instrument, body part, government agency
pack	small parcel, facial treatment, bundle, group of animals, association of criminals, to treat a body part, arrange in a container

page	knight's attendant, errand runner, call out someone's name, paper in a book
palm	inner hand, tree, touch with the hand
panel	sheet that forms a section, pad under a saddle, group of people gathered to plan or discuss, graphic user interface, electric device
pants	clothing, gasping for air
park	a recreational green space, to stop a car in a particular place, car gear
part	less than all, less than whole, line where hair is divided, portion, acting role, individual efforts, discontinue an association
pass	throwing a ball, aircraft flight, football play, free ticket, permit to enter, complete cycle, leave of absence, success in a test, brief attempt, allow to go uncensored, go across or through
patient	person requiring medical care, enduring without protest, even tempered
pen	writing tool, to write, enclosure for animals, jail, female swan
perch	to sit, fish, support that serves as a resting spot
period	punctuation mark, the end of something, distinct phase in life, unit of time
permit	legal document, formal authorization, allow the presence of, make possible
pet	domesticated animal, loved one, favorite, to stroke
physical	dealing with matter and energy, having material existence, involving the body, using force, complete medical examination
pick	basketball maneuver, heavy tool, device to pluck an instrument, a person chosen, best of a group, choosing, gather, provoke, remove in small bits
pinch	squeeze with fingers, painful circumstances, small amount, make off with belongings of others
pit	quarry, concealed trap, sizeable whole, area in front of a stage, inner layer of fruits, set into rivalry, mark with a scar

pitch	throwing something, card game, golf shot, property of sound, degree of deviation from horizontal, up and down motion, promotion by demonstration, erect and fasten
pitcher	position in baseball, container for liquids
place	particular location, slang for house or apartment, to set something down
plain	tract of land, lacking ornamentation, free from disguise, comprehensible to the general public, not mixed with anything
plane	tool, aircraft, unbounded two dimensional shape, level of existence
plant	living organism, building for industry, something hidden, an actor in an audience, put firmly in the mind, put seeds in the ground, lay the groundwork for, set securely
plate	dish, metal sheathing, receptacle for church collection, dental appliance, baseball equipment, coat with a layer of metal
play	fun activity, preset plan of action in sports, performance by actors, attempt to get something, space for movement, verbal wit, deliberate coordinated movement, to have an effect on
plot	a scheme, story line, chart showing progress, small area of ground
poach	cooking technique, hunt illegally
point	sharp end, outstanding characteristic, geometric element, object of an activity, brief version, unit of counting the score in sports, linear unit
poker	card game, fire iron
pole	long rod, sports implement, point when the earth's axis of rotation intersects with its surface
pool	game, excavation filled with water, organization of shared resources, small body of standing water, combination of funds
pop	sharp sound, sweet drink, type of music, informal word for *dad*, bulge outward
port	an opening, wine, place where people enter or leave a country, computer circuit, left side of a ship or aircraft, land or reach a point
position	job, assignment in sports, spatial property, arrangement of the body, a way of regarding topics, customary location, item in sequence, a condition in which you find yourself
positive	characterized by affirmation, number greater than zero, indicating existence, optimistic state of mind, impossible to deny
post	delivery and collection of letters, pole or stake set up to mark something, a job in an organization, to transfer entries, display, coming after
pound	unit of measurement, public enclosure for stray dogs, hit hard, foreign unit of money
press	to push, lift weights, printing machine, clamp, printed matter, state of urgency, to smooth clothes
prime	math term, time of maturity when power is the greatest, cover with a coat of paint, at the best stage
prop	support, moveable item on a movie set, propeller
prune	dried plum, weed out, to clip
punch	a blow with the fist, tool, beverage, to make a hole
pupil	student, eye part
purse	bag for carrying money, money offered as a prize, contract lips
quack	duck sound, untrained person who pretends to be a doctor
quality	distinguishing attribute, degree of excellence, a characteristic property, high social status, superior grade
quarter	district of a city, U.S. coin, division of a compass, one fourth, three months, division of the school year, fifteen minutes, execution method, a period of playing time in a sports contest
race	contest of speed, competition, division of species, to work fast, cause to move fast

Copyright © 2003 LinguiSystems, Inc.

racket	illegal enterprise, tennis equipment, loud noise
range	place for shooting or driving, variety of different things, limits of motion, open land, series of hills or mountains, kitchen appliance
rare	low density, uncommon, meat cooked a short time, not reoccurring often
rash	series of occurrences, red eruption of the skin, disregard for danger, to act without thinking
rate	charge relative to some basis, time unit, speed of process, be worthy of, assign a rank to, estimate the value
rattle	part of a snake's tail; baby toy; short, loud sounds
rear	side that goes last, farthest from the back, the hind part of a human or an animal, to raise
record	list of recognized accomplishments, extreme attainment, compilation of known facts, permanent evidence, wins vs. losses, sound recording
reflect	cast light, give evidence of quality, bend backward, think deeply
refrain	part of a song, not to do something,
relish	experience, savory condiment, get enjoyment from
report	short account of the new, inform verbally, written document, student's written evaluation, make known to the authorities, make a charge against
rest	freedom from activity, support, musical notation, death, items left after other parts have been taken away
rich	of great worth, pleasantly full and mellow, containing large amounts of choice ingredients, abundant supply of desirable qualities or substances, possessing material wealth
right	principles of justice, direction, conservative political orientation, make amends for, regain proper position, make correct, appropriate for the condition, free from error, socially correct, immediately, interjection expressing agreement

ring	circular band of jewelry, platform for wrestling or boxing, characteristic sound, association of criminals, circle
roast	piece of meat, negative criticism, cook with dry heat, to be hot
rock	pitch from side to side, mineral matter, candy, type of music
room	an area enclosed by walls, space for movement, opportunity for
rose	flower, color
round	circular, series of professional calls, ammunition, outburst of applause, cut of beef, serving for everyone, golf term, approximate to the nearest designated number
row	continuous succession without interruption, objects or people arranged in a line, linear array of numbers, sport, propel with oars, angry dispute
ruler	person who commands, measuring stick
run	score made in baseball, traveling on foot at a fast pace, a regular trip, a short trip, football play, unraveled stitches, deal in illegally, set animals to graze, make without a miss, execute a program or process
rung	cross piece on a chair, ladder part
runner	device on which things can slide, person employed to deliver messages, a person who travels on foot quickly, horizontal branch of a plant that produces new plants, a person who imports or exports without paying duties
safe	strongbox for valuables, free from danger, in good hands, financially sound
sage	herb, wise mentor, color
saw	tool, to cut, to have seen
scale	body part of fish, indicator, measuring instrument, relative magnitude, ratio between size and representation, ordered reference standard, to remove, reach the highest point, to cut back
school	group of fish, building of education, being formally educated, train to be discriminating

seal	marine animal, impression device, fastener, a finishing coat, approved superior status, make tight
season	period of the year, recurrent holiday time, lend flavor to, make fit
second	unit of time, following first, baseball term, to agree with a motion, imperfect merchandise, gear in a car
select	to choose, superior grade
sentence	string of words, prison time, final judgement
set	exercises done in a series, putting something in position, electronic equipment, decent of the sun, a group of things, abstract collections of numbers, unit of play in tennis, scenery in a production, permanent inclination, becoming hard, establish a record, ready to start a race
shake	grasp a person's hand, building material, reflex caused by cold, frothy ice-cream drink, undermine, get rid of, stir the feelings of
share	assets contributed, stock, individual efforts in a common goal, use jointly, communicate
sharp	musical note, pointed, keenly felt, quick and forceful, in great amount, harsh, bitter in taste
shed	an outbuilding, cast off hair, get rid of, pour out in drops
sheet	bed linen, piece of paper, flat thin material, to rain hard
shock	unpleasant surprise, bushy mass, grain set on ends to dry, bodily collapse, car part, feeling of distress, passage of electronic current

Page 149

shop	place of business, to browse, to compare
short	baseball term, electrical circuit problem, cheat someone, low in stature, most direct, having little length, speech sounds, direct

shot	attempt, immunization, attempt to score in a game, bullet from a gun, track equipment, hard blow to the body
sight	optical instrument, range of vision, ability to see, visual perception
sign	indication, written message, gesture to communicate, evidence, parts of the Zodiac, written agreement, to write your name
sink	plumbing fixture, descend into, golf term, go under
slide	gliding, transparency, rectangular plate, sloping chute, large mass of earth falling, baseball maneuver
slip	undergarment, to avoid capture, minor mistake, small piece of paper, accidental misstep, slender person, unexpected slide, part of a plant, get worse, boat dock
slug	insect, to hit hard, an idle person
snap	putting a football in play, fastener, easy activity, break suddenly, angry tone, sound made with fingers, record on film, grab hastily
soil	to get dirty, dirt
sole	fish, bottom of shoe or foot
solution	mixture, answer to a problem
sound	auditory effect, ocean inlet, cause to make noise, appear interesting, financially safe, excellent condition, morally correct, deeply, showing good judgment
space	expanse where everything is located, blank area, spot in line
spade	tool, suit in cards
spare	bowling term, an extra item, not needed, refrain from harming, relieve from experiencing, use frugally
speaker	someone who addresses a group, presiding officer, amplification device
spell	verbal formula, period of time, indicates, write or name the letters that form a word
spoke	wire support within a wheel, to have talked

spot	entertainment establishment, contrasting part of something, section assigned to a performer, small quantity, blemish, catch sight of
spring	spiral device, natural flow of water, season, elasticity of something, disclose suddenly, move forward quickly
square	tool, shape, old-fashioned, product of two equal terms, honesty, firmly, in a direct way
squash	a game, vegetable, compress
stable	farm building, dependable, maintaining equilibrium, showing little change
staff	strong rod, system that musical notes are written on, group of employees
stage	section or portion, large platform, the theatre as a profession, large coach with horses, time period, plan an event
stalk	threatening gait, hunt for game, slender structure, harass
stall	to put off, place within a barn for livestock, a stopped engine
stamp	a block used to imprint, token for paid postal fees, distinctive form, extinguish
stand	to be in an upright position, to be in a specified state, a booth with items for sale, defensive effort
staple	paper fastener, necessary item, to fasten
star	celestial body, a graphic design, an outstanding or famous person
state	the way something is, organized body of people, territory, express an idea
stay	remaining in a place, nautical brace, thin strip used to stiffen a garment, judicial order
steer	bull, direct the course, guiding force
stick	length of wood, pierce or puncture, cause to protrude, stay put, piece of hockey equipment, piece of gum
still	apparatus for making alcohol, static photograph, tranquil silence, cause to be quiet, free from current, absence of sound

stock	merchandise in a shop, lumber, capital raised by a corporation, descendants of an individual, supply for future use
strain	exertion, injury to muscle, nervousness from stress, group of organisms, force to the limit
strand	piece of complex fibers, necklace, abandon
straw	thin plastic tube, plant fiber, yellow color
strike	baseball pitch, bowling term, an attack, refusal to work, gentle blow, remove by erasing
strip	to undress, narrow flat piece of material, sequence of cartoon drawings, an airfield, to remove a covering from
stroke	light touch of the hand, single complete movement, to hit a golf ball, a mark made by writing, sudden loss of consciousness, treat gingerly
stump	part of a limb or tooth, base of a tree, cause to be perplexed
sty	pigpen, infection of the eye
submarine	submersible warship, sandwich
suspect	someone under suspicion, to believe a person is guilty, imagine to be true, regard as untrustworthy
swallow	bird, small amount of food or liquid, believe without questioning, to ingest food or drink
switch	changing for another, basketball maneuver, instrument of punishment, control device, railroad track device, one thing substituted for another, reverse
tag	a children's game, touching someone, a label, baseball term, provide with a nickname
tail	animal part, rear of an aircraft, a spy, last part of something, follow closely behind
tank	container, military vehicle, prison cell
tap	light touch, cutting tool, dancing shoe, faucet, draw from, furnish with a spigot

tape	long strip used for fastening, musical recording, line strung across the finishing point in a race
temple	place of worship, side of forehead
tense	category of verbs, stretch tightly, uncomfortable
tick	parasite, light mattress, tapping sound
tie	cord of material, horizontal beam, cross braces on a railroad track, equal score, neckwear, social or business relationship, to knot
tip	potential opportunity, extreme end, small amount of money for services, cause to tilt, to walk on your toes
tire	hoop that covers a wheel, exhaust through overuse, cause to be bored
toast	bread that has been browned, kind words before a drink, make brown and crisp
toll	fee levied, value measured, ring recurrently
top	clothing, covering for a hole, toy, greatest possible intensity, uppermost of anything, first half of an inning, canvas tent, to go beyond or better
toy	nonfunctional replica, breed of small dog, plaything, manipulate
track	sport, bars of rolled steel, evidence pointing to a solution, selection of music, racecourse, carry on the feet and deposit, to go after
trail	path, mark left by something, evidence pointing to a solution, proceed slowly, linger behind, to go after
train	public transportation, cloth on the back of a gown, a procession, force to grow in a certain way, undergo instruction, exercise to prepare for an event
truck	vehicle, hand cart, to transport, to move quickly
trunk	luggage, main stem of a tree, elephant's nose, torso, compartment in a car
tumbler	glassware, part of a lock, gymnast
tune	succession of notes, to adjust
turkey	bird, an event that fails badly, annoying or unpleasant person, three strikes in a row in bowling
turn	moving in the opposite direction, agreed succession, a favor, unforeseen development, become older, assume new characteristics, direct at someone, alter the function, pass into a condition, to let go
type	printed characters, a particular kind of thing, write with a keyboard
uniform	clothes with distinctive design for identification, evenly spaced, the same
utter	express audibly, extreme
vault	arched ceiling or roof, burial chamber, compartment for safekeeping valuables, leap over, gymnastic equipment
vice	moral weakness, division in police department
wake	a vigil, wave behind a boat, consequences of an event, be alert, stop sleeping
watch	to guard, portable timepiece, follow with eyes or mind, look attentively, to be on guard
wave	movement of water, hairdo, signaling with the hand, progressive disturbance
well	a hole dug to obtain water, enclosed compartment, come up, good health, high probability, satisfactory, suitably, financial comfort, extent or degree, intimate knowledge
whip	quick snap, instrument for hitting, thrash about, defeat thoroughly
will	persistent intent, legal document, decree or ordain
yard	enclosure for animals, land around a house, area for storage of cars, unit of length

1-10-9876

Copyright © 2003 LinguiSystems, Inc.